"*African American Magick* by Stephanie Rose Bird anoints us with seasonal rites encouraging people of color to honor their magick with open arms and a purposeful soul. As each chapter unfolds, Black magick becomes a blessed offering, a tapestry of traditional practices both native and foreign, a harmonizing truth within this spiritual ecosystem we call America. Stephanie's words shout, we are here and brought our Gods and Goddesses, our juju and lwas. We are here conjuring a stew of delicious folklore forever etched within our DNA. May you, as have I, devour each and every word to the bone."

—Mawiyah Kai EL-Jamah Bomani,
author of *Conjuring the Calabash: Empowering
Women with Hoodoo Spells and Magick*

"As a Priestess of Shango and Osain, it is very refreshing to see an 'Osayin Tea Party' woven into the landscape of this powerhouse African medley. Stephanie Rose Bird has blessed me and the entire world with this beautifully orchestrated grimoire that reflects the African American experience in her rarest and most treasured forms. This collection reads like a sweet lullaby to my soul. Thank you, Sacred Sister, for keeping our greatness alive!"

—Iya Angelique "Sobande" Greer,
master herbalist, holistic nutritionist, visionary founder of Sacred
Waters Retreat and the NCB School of Herbalism & Holistic Health

"Stephanie Rose Bird's mastery as an herbalist and skilled magickal practitioner shines through the pages of *African American Magick*. Brimming with recipes, rites, and herbal remedies, as well as a comprehensive appendix, that highlight her personal African American experiences, this book is an encyclopedia of spiritual guidance. It is a grimoire to return to again and again, as one navigates the wheel of life seeking practical, magickal ways to help heal and uplift mind, body, and soul."

—**Najah Lightfoot,** author of *Good Juju: Mojos, Rites & Practices for the Magical Soul* and *Powerful Juju: Goddesses, Music & Magic for Comfort, Guidance & Protection*

"Stephanie Rose Bird's inclusion of various paths and traditions with indigenous roots makes *African American Magick* a much needed and educational book. Living in Michigan, I tend to do certain rituals, rites, and practices with the seasons, and Bird provides seasonal workings. *African American Magick* is a must-have addition to your spiritual practice and book collection."

—**Yvette Wyatt,** owner of The MotownWitch

"African American Magick: A Modern Grimoire for the Natural Home by Stephanie Rose Bird is a book whose time has come! Using the bones of its earlier iteration as a foundation, this guide brings us into the present, acknowledging the impacts of global health traumas on our communities and the increased shift in our focus to *how* we care for ourselves, our families, and our homes. *African American Magick* is a grimoire that invites each reader to build on it, creating their own unique collection of recorded histories and practices for use now and as a 'gift from the ancestors' for future generations."

—**Rhonda Alin,** founder of Black Women of Magick & Conjure and founder of Northern New Jersey Tarot

"The brilliant Stephanie Rose Bird does it again! 'It' being uplifting the spiritual ingenuity of indigenous African spiritual practices. Bird lets us into her personal grimoires, giving us a look at the years of magic and experience she wields and possesses. She offers us a piece of her asè as she strengthens ours."

—**Empress Karen M. Rose,** author of *The Art and Practice of Spiritual Herbalism*

African American
MAGICK

➣ A Modern Grimoire for the Natural Home ⬿

STEPHANIE ROSE BIRD

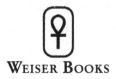

WEISER BOOKS

This edition first published in 2023 by Weiser Books,
an imprint of Red Wheel/Weiser, LLC
With offices at:
65 Parker Street, Suite 7
Newburyport, MA 01950
www.redwheelweiser.com

Some sections of this book appeared previously in article form in *Natural Home and Garden
Magazine* and *NaturallyCurly.com*. Permission has been granted to incorporate this material.
Species-At-Risk compiled by United Plant Savers, a nonprofit education corporation
dedicated to preserving native medicinal plants, used by permission.

ISBN: 978-1-57863-784-3

Library of Congress Cataloging-in-Publication Data

Names: Bird, Stephanie Rose, 1960- author.
Title: African American magick : a modern grimoire for the natural home /
   Stephanie Rose Bird.
Description: Newburyport, MA : Weiser Books, an imprint of Red
   Wheel/Weiser, LLC, 2023. | Includes bibliographical references and
   index. | Summary: "African American Magick infuses ancient techniques,
   rituals, and methods from around the world to use each season's inherent
   energies to supplement the health and well-being of body, mind, and
   soul. The changing of the seasons can feel magical - greens changing to
   browns and golds, snow melting to show fresh buds. We all recognize
   these telltale signs, but few of us are aware of the powerful impact
   each season has on our spiritual lives. In African American Magick,
   Stephanie Rose Bird infuses ancient techniques, rituals, and methods
   from around the world to use each season's inherent energies to
   supplement body, mind, and soul. Designed to further spiritual practices
   by learning from neighboring cultures, this book provides readers with
   useful ideas unrestricted by geographic borders, ethnicity, religion, or
   magical path. Included are recipes and concepts from the Caribbean,
   African American soul food, Buddhist meditation practices, sacred Hindu
   rites, Old European traditions, Australian Aboriginal dreaming lessons,
   and Native American wisdom "-- Provided by publisher.
Identifiers: LCCN 2022059739 | ISBN 9781578637843 (trade paperback) | ISBN
   9781633412736 (kindle edition)
Subjects: LCSH: African American magic. | Naturopathy. | BISAC: BODY, MIND
   & SPIRIT / Magick Studies | RELIGION / Indigenous, Folk & Tribal
Classification: LCC BF1622.A34 B565 2023 | DDC 615.5/35--dc23/eng/20230202
LC record available at https://lccn.loc.gov/2022059739

Cover design by Sky Peck Design
Interior by Steve Amarillo / Urban Design LLC
Typeset in Adobe Minion and Avenir Next

Printed in the United States of America
IBI
10 9 8 7 6 5 4 3 2 1

*For the Warramirri (People Who Own the Red Cloud)
of Galiwin'ku, Elcho Island in the Northern Territory
and the people at the outstation of Maparu in Australia
who kindly adopted my family into theirs and showed
us how the ancient ways continue in the modern day.*

*Six thousand years and still going; may
fair winds blow upon you always.*

Blessed Be!

Contents

Winter

Spring

Summer

Autumn

Acknowledgments

I am humbled by the grace of Mother Nature and awestricken by her omnipresence and power. I wish to thank my ancestors and relatives for shaping and forming my being. I am grateful to my family, husband, children and their partners for their love, support, and inspiration. I want to extend a special thanks to my personal editor Jannette Giles for helping me all along the way of this magical journey. I appreciate the belief in this project, support, and assistance from the beautiful spirits at Weiser Books for resurrecting this popular seasonal guide, including,

Peter Turner, Weiser Books associate publisher; Jane Hagaman, managing editor; and my dear friend and fellow Magickmaker Judika Illes. A big thanks also to copyeditor Rachel Nagengast and Marketing manager Gia Manalio-Bonaventura. I deeply appreciate the incredible contribution of Kathryn Sky-Peck for powerful and visionary cover art and design. May many blessings and wonderful mojo blow toward the Motherland, the fair isles of the Caribbean, North and South Americas and elsewhere in the African diaspora. Ashe!

Blessed Be!

Preface

Two years after my first book, *Sticks, Stones, Roots and Bones: Hoodoo, Mojo and Conjuring with Herbs,* was published came my second book. Back in 2006, *Four Seasons of Mojo: An Herbal Guide to Natural Living* came along. The main thrust of *Four Seasons of Mojo* was to help readers take the almost inexplicable power and mystery of that energizing force referred to as mojo and utilize it in the way we live, with intention. Along with herbs, that precious gift of Mama Nature, the book took readers on a magickal journey into what was then a very different way of life—one that was in lock-step with the unique rhythms of nature, called simply, natural living. Today, Blessed Be!, green living and natural living is second nature to many. This gladdens my heart. However, there are still many more who are either curious or taking the first steps on the path to natural living.

After the upheaval to the mind, body, and spirit evoked by the COVID-19 pandemic, all manner of folk are in search of natural options for healing and wellness. Many are turning back to the soil and exploring herbs to treat a wide variety of ills. Some work from home and find that they have more time for juicing, canning, freezing, making, and using herbal soaps, floor washes, tinctures, tisanes, and other herbal preparations.

COVID-19, in its many guises and strands, is still with us, as is the uneasiness, and in some cases, darkness that it has brought with it. In herbal guides from around the world, there are medicines to be found that are antibacterial, antimicrobial, immunity-building, antidepressant, antianxiety, sleep promoting, and relaxing. These earth medicines come from trees—their bark, pods, roots, leaves, and flowers—as well as plants and herbs that we can engage with in order to achieve better mental and physical health in addition to good hygiene.

So, it is with great pleasure that I announce my *Four Seasons of Mojo* has been revived and is now re-presented to the enquiring mind by Weiser Books. Hats off also to the book's illustrator for a breathtaking cover image that so clearly encapsulates the words, thoughts, and themes being put forth in what is now called *African American Magick: A Modern Grimoire for the Natural Home*. Through the four seasons of recipes, herbs, and rituals in these pages, we envision the new title— *African American Magick*, a subject which we need to delve into further here, before you get started in the larger body of the text.

There is a complex, rich, and vast corpus of knowledge within the topic of African American magick. It cannot be painted with a broad brush. Through lived experience, ancestral stories, and the legacy built on precious memories, each of us, whether reader, practitioner, author, or any combination of the above, bring original thoughts and interpretations of African American magick. The folklore, traditions, mythology, spirituality, and healing ways of black people is held in the hands of our diaspora, to hold close or share as we see fit.

Some of the magick of this book comes from the number four of the elements, which are employed in the work, as well as the seasons and major life passages. This book frames its contribution to the understanding of African American magick with a specific setting—the home. In the home, the practical, also referred to as mundane, and the spiritual, which may also be sacred, merge. As you turn these pages physically or metaphorically, experiencing its mélange of *ashe*, seasonal magick, life passages, and matters of the home an enrichment in the form of a grimoire manifests.

Since practicing herbalism, aromatherapy, and magick-making of various types, I have found the grimoire to be an essential tool. It is also an extension of my magick-making. The grimoire is ancient and contemporary, now and later, like the *lwas* of Haiti and the dreamings of Australia. It holds an ever-living, evolving history. The grimoire shapes and molds, while capturing what may someday be legacy. Therefore, the subtitle of this book—*A Modern Grimoire for the Natural Home*—is important.

Though there are elements of history, ancestry, and legacy embodied and shared, this and all my books thrive on the concept of modernity. Their contemporary spirit will inevitably shine through because they are not carefully crafted regurgitations; instead they are built on interpretation and deep thought.

As you enter this text, bring an open and curious heart and mind. Through your openness and curiosity, combined with your willingness to experiment and try new things the reader experience expands. By taking notes in your own grimoire, which can be a book, as simple or fancy as you'd like it to be, the corpus expands and stays alive. Together, we the people of the African diaspora make African American magick what it is. *African American Magick* is one of my contributions to this knowledge base. Read, absorb, experiment, try things, let what you need in, as you live your best green life in step with Mama Nature.

Ashe and Green Blessings!

—Stephanie Rose Bird

CHAPTER ONE

The Magic and Mystery of the Seasons

African American Magick: A Modern Grimoire for the Natural Home examines the magical ability of the seasons to enhance our lives. Like most of my work, this book honors the old ways of the earth's original people as well as their descendants, the people of Africa, the Caribbean, and Americas. We go further afield to learn from neighboring cultures; people with influential magical practices derived from living close to the earth. As a practicing Hoodoo, I honor eclecticism. I have designed *African American Magick* to provide readers with useful ideas unrestricted by geographic borders, ethnicity, religion, or magical path. Within these pages you will find delightful recipes from the Caribbean, soul food of African Americans, meditation practices of Buddhists, Hindu rites, the ways of Old Europe, and lessons of the Australian Aboriginal dreaming and Native American traditions alike.

Whether sunny, snowy, windy, rainy, cold, or humid, the weather has a dramatic effect on our lives wherever we may live. In Africa, duality is a very important phenomenon. The year is divided into two opposing weather conditions called the wet and the dry. The dry is a time when life is most challenged, and resources literally dry up. Water, the most cherished elixir of life, is hard for animals, humans, and plants to find. The wet is joyous but it has challenges of its own. The joy comes from the first rains of the season because these bring with them sustenance—the rains ensure the continuance of life. The interaction between earth and the heavens is heightened. Rock-hard soil becomes malleable enough to make mud, useful as a health and beauty remedy as well as a source for constructing unique round houses.

If the rains continue for weeks unabated, there is concern of floods with their accompanying disruptions. Floods wash out dams, enhancing destruction. Other infrastructures critical to modern life such as roads and bridges may also be damaged or destroyed by floods. Livestock, wild animals, food crops, and wild foods are frequently impacted, threatening the livelihood and sustenance of entire communities. For nomadic people, rains are especially challenging because often there is a lack of overhead shelter; they are truly at the whim of the elements.

In the United States, many people have become distanced from the seasons. For the most part in the West, weather is looked upon as a temporary nuisance, reported by a weatherperson rather than being directly observed by the seers of the immediate community. In the States, weather is a "condition" to be treated almost like a medical illness, with a variety of electronics or protective gadgets. Whereas the wet season in Africa and many other locales is a time for celebration, here rain is something that threatens our outdoor events, or more trivial still, causes frizzy hair. Only when we have droughts and our lovely flowers or endless green lawns are dried to a frizzled brown do we tend to take heed of rain or the lack thereof.

On the other side of the coin are people intensely interested in the seasons and their relationship to the bottom line—these folks include marketing analysts and business people in a variety of other commercial enterprises. It is a sad reality that most of the agrarian celebrations that have survived to the present day have only been kept alive because they afford an opportunity to make money from the mass marketing of food, gifts, and costly indulgence. For instance, Samhain and All Hallows' Eve have grown into modern Halloween, and Yule has grown into modern-day Christmas.

African American Magick takes an alternate view of the seasons and the powerful impact they can have in our lives. This book instills the importance of each quarter of our year on our health. I share seasonal traditions that can be adapted and utilized to infuse holistic health into the mind, body, and spirit. *African American Magick* takes a fresh look at the seasons and the weather conditions they inspire, putting you in touch with the ways in which the heavens are important to this earth.

Solstice and the Equinox

Our modern term "season" really refers to a period of the year that begins with one of two astronomical bi-annual occurrences—the solstice or the equinox. While it is enjoying wider use in large part due to the earth-based spirituality movement that embraces the traditions of our ancestors, most people still don't know what the solstices are or how they differ from the equinoxes. If you could visualize the year as a circle, similar to a wheel rather than in the linear fashion of our modern-day calendars, you will take a step closer to understanding the concept on which our seasons are built. I like to take it a step further and visualize the year as a delectable pie. Take that pie, slice it into four equal segments and you have the four seasons of the year, also known as the quarter days, marked by celebrations and rites.

The solstices create two of those important slices of our year and they oppose one another within the circle. The word solstice translates to "sun standing still." They are the points during Earth's orbit when our hemisphere is closest to or farthest from the Sun. For example, the summer solstice occurs around June 22 of each year. The Sun enters Cancer at 23.5 degrees N declination and in relation to us in the northern hemisphere our star reaches its highest point, for it is situated directly above us. Our other solstice is the winter solstice, which occurs around December 21 annually.

The Igbo, a group of Africans concentrated in Nigeria, have a corpus of ancient knowledge that is very involved with keeping and marking time as well as with astrology. The wise people of the Igbo are called Dibia. John Anenechukwu Umeh has graced us with some of the secrets of their cosmology. Within his book *After God is Dibia, Vol. 2* he explains solstice and equinox from the perspective of his people. This perspective speaks of a tilting, described by the Igbo as:

Obi aha-ada ada (aha-ada gwo m) o na-abu o daita ogbukelu egbukelu o ga-eji binitekwa na oge/mgbe di n'chu.[1]

This is translated roughly, "The obi sacred house does not fall flat or outright. It falls partially and stabilizes in a tilt, which posture would enable it to spring up again in due course." In other words, the wheel of the year continues to move and with it the seasons will always change. Dibia mark this sentiment with charms, rituals, and sometimes sacrifices.

Even in tropical Africa there is a winter, albeit not as dramatic as in other places. The Igbo call it *Ugulu,* meaning "a little winter." Winter and summer solstice are celebrated in various parts of Africa just as they are celebrated across the world by people who live close to the earth, be they nomadic or agrarian societies.

There are two other times of great importance in Africa that are important elsewhere on our planet—they are the two equinoxes. The daylight hours, that precious time when we get most of our work done, are impacted by the equinoxes, those times when day and night enjoy a balanced relationship. In Africa, the equinoxes are observed in subtle ceremony and rites. The word equinox means equal night. The first equinox occurs when the Sun enters Aries; this is called the vernal equinox, known popularly as spring. The second equinox occurs when the Sun enters Libra; this event marks the beginning of fall, also called the autumnal equinox. The solstices are useful dividing points in the year, giving us three months each of winter, spring, summer, and fall.

Different cultures have used various means of dividing the year and marking the seasons. One of the more colorful ways is by naming the moons of each month. For example, in the United States there are numerous names for the different moons of each month. The Native American nations have one of the most in-depth ways of matching up the moons with seasonal weather conditions and the various stages of plant growth, encompassing planting times, weeding, the various harvests of specific plants, and when the ground rests. The Native

American moons also observe the activities of the animals, weather, and conditions in the sky. There is no single naming, as each nation has its own vital traditions, and obviously the weather, flora, and fauna change quite dramatically across North America.

The Celtic people had an equally enchanting method of marking the months using trees and sometimes other plants such as reeds. This system of observing the year stems from the Celtic tradition of tree veneration. Today people are keeping the Celtic ways alive and the tree months continue to be observed. Some people in the United States have merged the Celtic system of understanding each month through the symbolism of trees with the Native American way of naming the moons. Rather than Celtic Tree Months this system has become more focused on moons, thus there are Celtic Tree Months such as Oak Moon, which we will explore later. *The Farmer's Almanac* uses a very eclectic system, drawing bits and pieces from various Native American nations and establishing its own way of marking time using the moons.

Within the pages of *African American Magick*, you will have the opportunity to engage in activities inspired by moon lore from Native American nations and from the Celtic tree traditions. This will encourage you to activate or deepen your understanding of the seasons by making connections between earth and sky.

Whether you celebrate Kwanzaa, the African American harvest festival of the first fruits, Chanukah, the festival of lights, Yule, the Pagan observance of the winter solstice which looks forward to the return of the Sun, or Christmas, the familiar Christian holiday that marks the birth of the Son of God, I'm sure most of you enjoy gifts emblematic of the season. This book is my gift to you. I have stocked *African American Magick* like a thoughtfully prepared mojo bag filled with magical ingredients. This is mojo designed to help you enjoy abundance and health year round. This book is devoted to presenting a variety of ways of living in accordance with nature. It is divided into quarters just like the pie I described, focused on winter, spring, summer, and fall, centering on the holidays of those seasons, coordinating with our calendar year.

Seasonal Mojo

Hoodoo is the magic that I frequently practice. Intimately entwined with Hoodoo, which is sometimes confusingly called Voodoo, is the term mojo. Before we get into mojo, let's discuss Hoodoo.

The word Hoodoo is useful for giving form to the colorful and specific folkloric beliefs practiced by a wide range of believers including the Gullah people of Georgia and the Carolinas, Black folk in major metropolitan areas, White folk of the Appalachians, and Native Americans. Hoodoo has always been practiced by a wide variety of people, regardless of ethnicity or religious affiliation—it is not a religion but a collection of folk practices involving magic and healing. Its attractiveness lies in the fact that it is natural, nondogmatic, and practical. Primary concerns include blessing the home and keeping the domestic environment peaceful and free of unwanted intrusions, whether they are bad vibes brought about by humans, animals, or spirits. Hoodoo is concerned with health, wealth, love, luck, and happiness—concerns with which many people can relate.

The means used to achieve a desired situation is called the "laying of tricks" or "fixing tricks," which is akin to European witchcraft spells and has roots in Romani charms. These objects are a New World adaptation of African herbal bundles. The most common form is a bag of tricks that employs herbs and other magical ingredients called nation sacks, gris-gris, hands, trick bags, luck balls, flannels, and most popularly, mojos. The use of the term "my mojo" and "his or her bag of tricks" is often included in the lyrics of traditional African American blues singers, particularly the legendary Muddy Waters, who is also called the Hoodoo Man. Unfortunately, the lyrics have been misinterpreted—mojo was interpreted as a metaphysical aura of sexual power or prowess, whereas the trick bag was misinterpreted as a metaphor for various forms of misleading behaviors. In reality, a mojo and a bag of tricks are one and the same—a bag of charms that serves as an amulet for purposes ranging from attracting a lover and maintaining a relationship to drawing luck or attracting money. The mojo bags are carried close to the person, usually on the thigh, in the bra, or in a special pouch under the clothing. If someone steals your mojo, they have stolen your special amulet that holds your hopes and dreams. The mojo is a personalized item that carries your personal energy; therefore, it could be very dangerous or even fatal for it to fall into the hands of another, especially if that person is a Hoodoo, witch, or conjurer.

Clearly, most Hoodoos would not like to see the word mojo used lightly, and I am using it with all its weight and power in the pages of this book. Mojo is a collective force that helps build personal power. It is the tool of the warrior and shaman, even in modern-day urban life. Controversy swirls around the origins of the word mojo. While doing research for my first book, *Sticks, Stones, Roots & Bones: Hoodoo, Mojo & Conjuring with Herbs*, I learned that the Bamana of the Western Sudan use power objects such as medicine bags that are imbued with ashe (life force energy) for addressing various ills. Warriors use these objects to express power. The bags are also used to fight supernatural malaise and to foil evil intentions. They contain *bilongo* (medicine) and a *mooyo* (soul). Mooyo and bilongo are West African predecessors of the word mojo, and these two words capture the spirit of mojo as we understand it in America—soul medicine. Soul medicine is the essence of mojo, and it forms the spiritual nexus of this book.

Mojo is a tool of the Hoodoo. Mojo bags are popular in the African American community, used very similarly to medicine bags or the healing pouch used in magical healing traditions by shamans, and healers from various cultures. A mojo is a bag full of charms of animal, plant, mineral, and yes, even weather event remnants like lightning-felled branches and rainwater. For example, it may contain a wishbone from a chicken for good luck, a High John the Conqueror root for strength and endurance, a pair of matched lodestones for attraction, a rose quartz for a loving heart, and a piece of wood from a tree felled by lightning for powerful energy. Together such ingredients become an enigmatic charm designed to empower its owner, giving them an invisible shield of protection, charisma, and force.

Speaking in Metaphorical Tongues

Just as often as it refers to a real power object, mojo is also used metaphorically to suggest force, power, or prowess. This book is designed to help you harness the multiple energies, power, force, and mystical spirit of African American magick. *African American Magick* addresses rites of passage while at the same time comparing each stage of life to its equivalent time of the calendar year.

I see this book as a collection of mojo, filled with holistic medicine derived from the seasons. *African American Magick* is neatly divided into the seasons many of us know so well. They are used only as a guideline, providing a frame of reference most people can relate to. Many of the projects and inspirations can be done at other times of the year for various situations, and depending on where you live.

A Modern Grimoire for the Natural Home

Just about every witch, wizard, or sorcerer keeps a grimoire. Fellow Green Witch and award-winning author Ann Moura recently wrote the most eloquent description I've seen on the meaning of grimoire. She describes her book *Grimoire for the Green Witch: A Complete Book of Shadows* as not being "your usual reading book but a tool meant to be picked up and used—much like a cookbook—without lengthy discussions, reminiscences, explanations, or even formal sentences." She describes the word grimoire as being "deliciously medieval," derived from the word "grammar," a primer covering a field of knowledge.[2]

When I consider the connection between "grammar" and "grimoire," I realize the importance of this ancient way of rendering knowledge. Grammar and the grimoire are two building blocks for our language and communications, enabling us to describe the ways we find meaning within our existence.

A grimoire is a document of life, akin to a journal, diary, or recipe book with a focus on magical and spiritual fulfillment. Grimoires usually contain spells, rituals, ceremonies, chants, incantations, recipes, formulae, and invocations. Like a cookbook, this grimoire teaches the readers to create soul foods to nourish the mind, body, and spirit. Soul food is part of the vernacular of my people that transcends filling the belly. It goes back to the notion of the bilongo and mooyo—it is soul medicine and a rich reservoir of our unique culture.

Grimoires are shaped by experience—experiences with our natural environment in various stages of the moon, parts of the year, and passages in life. These special documents are valuable resources that guide us through a variety of situations, allowing us to help others and ourselves. Moreover, grimoires are based largely around a relationship with Mother Nature and have a relationship with ancient ways. Within their pages you can learn the qualities of various herbs, fruits, vegetables, minerals, stones, and animals. The recipes, incantations, practices, and spells contained herein are taken directly from my collections of grimoires.

The Natural Home

My first book, *Sticks, Stones, Roots and Bones: Hoodoo, Mojo and Conjuring with Herbs,* was written as a guide for Hoodoos, crafted around the notion of mojo as a power object. *African American Magick* differs from my first book by focusing most of its energy on our most intimate space, the home environment, and it is devoted almost entirely to holistic health. As an herbalist and aromatherapist, my emphasis is always on natural, earth-wise solutions to mundane as well as spiritual issues. *African American Magick* is designed to help imbue your home with natural energy that is truly magical. It is a transformative energy courtesy of Mother Nature's four seasons. This book stresses beauty cultivated through holistic health with a special focus on the herbal spirituality that is a hallmark of many African cultures. Harnessing this energy will fill your life with positive mojo.

A Final Word to the Wise

Remember what I say in all my work: if you do not have everything required to fulfill a recipe, make do by substituting what you have for what is required. As long as you don't substitute the key ingredients, the recipes should still work well. This also goes for the rituals, ceremonies, and other inspirations provided.

We begin our work with winter because I live in a temperate zone with four distinct seasons. For those who live elsewhere, where there is only the wet and the dry for example, you can use my spring and summer inspirations for the wet and the autumn and winter sections for your dry season. Enjoy the journey!

CHAPTER TWO

Elbow Grease

Tools and Equipment for Working Roots

The Means of Working Roots

Before we delve into the recipes and rituals, it is important to know what is required. This chapter features suggestions for the tools, equipment, and ways of working herbs by providing practical hands-on information. The beauty of African-inspired herbalism is that it incorporates the best of both worlds—East and West come together, melding medicine with magical intent capable of touching the spirit realm.

In the next few pages there is a listing of some of the most useful tools to help you in the journey toward practicing rootwork—some of these ways and means will seem very African, whereas others will seem more Western. However you slice it, these tools will enable you to carry forward the projects presented in the coming chapters.

Tools

Baskets: preferably made of sweetgrass or other hand-woven natural material for harvesting and for holding freshly harvested fruits, vegetables, and herbs. Sweetgrass baskets are made primarily by the Gullah people and sold at markets in Charleston, South Carolina and other Low Country, seacoast island locations. Some sweetgrass basket co-ops now also make these available online at virtual stores.

Blender: glass or stainless steel pitcher preferred over plastic because they can be thoroughly cleansed, whereas some residual matter may be retained in plastic, contaminating future blends. Blenders are used for thorough mixing and liquefying of a variety of natural ingredients including vegetables, fruits, and grains.

Bottles and jars: are very important pieces of equipment. I like using recycled bottles as much as possible to store homemade shampoo and conditioners. Mouthwash bottles, liquid dish detergent, shampoo and conditioner bottles as well as lotion, yogurt, and baby food containers are all useful. At times you will want to make special blends as gifts or for stores. There are plenty of specialty containers suppliers who carry powder dispensers, spray-topped bottles, cologne bottles, flip-top body wash bottles, and decorative jars with screw tops for this purpose. It's nice now and again to use decorative containers for yourself, especially the powder dispensers, since powders are important to African herbalism. Remember that when using recycled materials it is very important to sterilize them first by boiling plastic containers and cleansing glass bottles with very hot soapy water; rinse and allow to dry before beginning. They can also be sterilized in a dishwasher if you have one.

Cauldron: this doesn't have to be fancy or bought from a specialty shop—a plain cast iron Dutch oven will do. However, if you want to brew your potions in a proper cauldron there are plenty of suppliers who carry them.

Charcoal blocks: buy these in quantity, as they are the most efficient way of burning loose herbal incense (avoid those that contain saltpeter—it is toxic when burned). Pure bamboo charcoals from Japan are available and make a more wholesome alternative.

Chimenea: a miniature fireplace which is portable and generally kept on the patio. This is great for burning incense and for fire rituals if you don't have a fireplace. These are growing in popularity, thus they are more widely available and are sometimes simply referred to as patio fireplaces. Look for these at garden centers, home renovation shops, sporting goods stores, and specialty shops.

Coffee bean grinder: an electric-powered tool with swiveling blades, the coffee bean grinder is a convenient way to grind tough spices and roots compared to its ancestor, the mortar and pestle, which requires hand grinding and lots of elbow grease. (Watch out, though: really tough spices and roots need to be ground by hand, or they'll break your coffee grinder—trust me, I've been through quite a few.) These are available at coffee shops, home improvement centers, department stores, and discount shops.

Double boiler: this is an indirect way of heating that prevents waxy mixtures like ointments and candle wax from cooking too quickly. A double boiler can be improvised by floating a stainless steel bowl in water in a pot slightly larger than the stainless steel bowl.

Droppers: are essential for dispensing droplets of essential oils and fragrance oils. In magical jobs involving Hoodoo, blood, semen, and saliva, as well as other body fluids may be dispensed using them. Throughout the book I ask that you drop in essential oils; this is the approach used by good perfumers, because it helps ensure that the oils don't clump up, instead they disperse evenly.

Drying rack: this is an implement on which fresh herbs are hung by their stems and left to dry. Also, an attractive way to display and store dried herbs indefinitely.

Freestanding mixer: a convenient but not essential tool. Used for whisking and thoroughly blending ingredients while saving your personal energy.

Food processor: even a mini model without all the fancy attachments will do to blend and liquefy ingredients for personal care recipes.

Funnel set: used to prevent spills and ease transfer of liquids, oils, and powders from the bowl or pan to a small-necked bottle, referred to here as bottling.

Glass storage jars: are used mainly for oil infusions and tinctures. Tinted glass jars with spring or cork tops work well. Don't forget to sterilize first.

Gloves: thick cloth to protect the hands when harvesting berries, rose hips, roses, or other thorny branches; plastic gloves to keep your hands from contaminating herbal infusions, brews, decoctions, balms, salts, or other handmade herbal blends.

Grater: Teflon or stainless steel graters are recommended because they last longer and resist sticking and rusting. Mainly used for shredding beeswax and refining roots.

Juicer: creates fruit and vegetable juices.

Kerchief: these are made of simple cloth, plain or patterned, and they come in handy for keeping your locs, braids, or any type of hairstyle away from your brews and blends. Some ingredients you work with are damaging to the hair and irritating to the scalp so it is good to protect your hair while working herbs. It is also important to maintain the highest standard of cleanliness possible so that your herbal blends, brews, or potions are less likely to become contaminated by bacteria, dirt, or oils.

Kettle: to heat water used for infusing herbs.

Measuring spoons: made of stainless steel with clearly marked measurements etched into the surface are preferred.

Mixing bowls: glass, ceramic, or stainless steel is recommended because they will not become stained from colorants, nor will they harbor bits of leftover ingredients once cleaned properly. Cleanliness is very important, because dirty bowls or other equipment will introduce bacteria to your recipes, lessening their longevity and efficacy.

Mortar and pestle: this is a hand-grinding tool set, consisting of a bowl and a stick-like grinding tool that can be made of wood, marble, soapstone, or various other materials. In many ways it is symbolic of the African community and it is an essential tool of both the cook and the healer. Quite frequently when the African village is depicted in African stele or other forms of art, the mortar and pestle is figured prominently because the set is considered an indispensable tool for sustenance. Mortars and pestles are used for food preparation, grinding flour from various grains to make bread, and most important to our discussion here, the mortar and pestle is used to hand grind resins, tough spices, barks, roots, berries, grasses, leaves, and flowers. I recommend hand grinding with a mortar and pestle over using a food processor or coffee bean grinder because the process allows the healer to become influenced by the healing spirit energy of the plant. The energy of the plant is released along with the aromatic oils of the plant that is being ground, diffusing this energy into the air, and imbuing the environment and your soul with force and power.

Nonreactive measuring cups: both dry and liquid types. Pyrex, tempered glass, and stainless steel work best. Glass and stainless steel measuring cups are easy to clean, thoroughly preventing cross-contamination of ingredients from remnants of herbs and other debris.

Plastic bags: to temporarily contain spices or other dried materials that require airtight storage.

Plastic caps: used for placing over head and hair to trap body heat and encourage penetration of conditioners and colorants, while keeping messy treatments off neck and clothing.

Pot holders: quite a bit of herbal work involves heat; pot holders protect your hands from burning and are essential when working with infusions, decoctions, and other brews dependent on heat.

Pruning shears: it is good to have a sharp pair of heavy-duty shears for harvesting woody herbs, plants like roses that have thorns, evergreen branches, and other tough materials.

Scissors: you will need to have scissors on hand for cutting twine, string, cheesecloth, and leaves.

Splash-proof apron: highly recommended protection against the caustic sodium hydroxide used during cold processed soapmaking. Also consider putting on old clothes to use as smocks or work clothes.

Stainless steel pans: with heavy bottoms work best because they distribute heat evenly and resist burning and over-heating. Most importantly, stainless steel stays inert which prevents contamination and depletion which are likely to occur while using cast iron, aluminum, or copper. Make sure you have tight-fitting lids handy as well because they help retain the medicinal qualities of the volatile oils. Otherwise, these precious substances evaporate. Stainless steel whisks and stirring spoons are recommended for the same reasons.

Stove or hotplate: for heating, drying, and simmering decoctions, potions, and brews.

Straining devices: can be cheesecloth (muslin) stretched over a preserve or other wide-necked jar and secured with rubber band, twine, or what I prefer to use, a stainless steel sieve.

Stirring wand: usually made of nonreactive glass or ceramic, used similarly to a cocktail stirrer to blend perfumes while discouraging cross-contamination.

Storage bins: used to hold dried herbs. Dark glass containers with spring tops or stainless steel are ideal. Keeping light away from the herbs helps them retain their medicinal qualities longer. Some folk store them in brown paper bags, particularly when they are being dried. This works well only if you don't have moths or other pests that might try to eat the herbs.

Sun tea jars: glass or plastic jars used to brew herbs in sun or moonlight.

Thermometers: candy thermometers will work, but a meat probe is my first choice, because it will not break as easily. Thermometers are essential for soapmaking and are useful for checking temperatures during the creation of creams, salves, and healing balms.

Twine: is good for tying herbs together at the stems before hanging them to dry and for fixing muslin to a jar for straining. Hemp (marijuana) string is an excellent alternative for strength and durability.

Ways of Rootworking: Freeing Up the Ashe

Once you have a good collection of tools, your means for rootworking, the fun is just about to start. *Ashe*—the liquid essence of a tree, plant, root, flower, bud, berry, or leaf that contains healing energy—can be collected in various ways. To capture this precious energy, try some of the following traditional herbalism methods:

Agbo (African infusion method): a vegetable or fruit (called *aseje*, meaning "medicinal food") or an herb is infused in water and then squeezed by hand to release the ashe.

Agunmu (Pounded Medicine): this is an herbal substance including resins that are powdered on a grinding stone.

Decoction: made by extracting ashe from the tougher parts of the plant including the roots, bark, or berries. Decoction is accomplished by simmering these parts in a covered pan of water over medium-low heat for thirty minutes to five hours depending on the toughness of the herb. Once this process is complete, the ashe is readily available for healing work in the brew, which is formally called a decoction.

Etu (Burnt Medicine): slowly charring ingredients in a heavy pot, typically made of cast iron. The etu is then consumed as is or used in a body rub.

Infusion: can be either water-based or oil-based. Water-based infusions are teas containing ashe, also called tisanes or brews. Infusions are made by extracting the volatile oils of a plant in the following manner: pour boiling distilled water over the herb, and keep it covered for thirty minutes to one hour. Heating in water for a longer time on a very low temperature on the stovetop infuses tougher herbs. The pot should be tightly covered to retain the healing medicine rather than allowing it to escape into the air.

Maceration: helps release the volatile oils and delicate scents of buds and flowers. To macerate buds, mash them up in a mortar with a pestle or pulse for thirty seconds in a mini food processor.

Oil-based infusion: extract the volatile oils from herbs by putting herbal materials into a sterilized (dry) container; fill the jar to the top with loosely packed dried herbs; pour on a preferred oil such as olive oil, sunflower oil, sweet almond oil, or safflower oil, covering the plants completely and filling the jar to the top. Cover tightly, keep away from direct sunlight, and give the jar a whirl every day for four to six weeks (depending on desired strength).

Tincture: the extraction of healing medicines from herbs created by using 100-proof alcohols such as vodka, grain alcohol, rum, or ethanol. The concentrations of volatile oils are greater in tinctures than through infusion or decoction. Procedure: a sterilized jar is filled to the top with loosely packed herbal material. Be sure to use alcohol like vodka (do not use rubbing alcohol; it is too harsh and it smells so strong that it will overpower any attempts at scenting). Place on a sunny windowsill and swirl gently every day for four to six weeks; strain off herbal material and pour into a sterilized tinted bottle. Cover with a cork or other tight-fitted top.

Specialties

Maceration: A substance similar to a tincture can be created by following this procedure but replacing the alcohol with different liquids. Vinegar makes an acidic extract. Macerated buds or flower petals added to vegetable glycerin make an emollient, scented extract; and honey poured over macerated buds or petals produces an edible emollient tincture that is delicately scented and terrific in love potions or in edible body rubs.

Magical Spirit Hand: Often the nondominant hand is used in preparation and consumption of magical or spiritual medicines. This hand is typically the left hand, considered the magical hand, as many people are right-handed. As a lefty, I might add a note to others like me that you would want to switch to your right hand if utilizing this technique, because that would be the special hand for you as it is not used in mundane activity.

Toddies: Since the ancient African civilizations at Axum, Kush, Nubia, Khemet, and Egypt, African healers have combined herbal infusions with wine or other alcoholic beverages.

Spirit Works within the Roots

Knowing the proper harvesting, drying, handling, and extracting techniques is essential to African herbalism, but it is by no means the last word. The term "workin' roots" means that you should try to incorporate affirmations, incantations, and prayers if you wish, or meditation as you work with herbs in order to access their spirit energy. The second half of this book features recipes combined with various types of magical work that will help you call up the ancestors or spiritual helpers to assist with healing.

Speaking directly to the pot, fire, candle, or herb is also essential. Remember that rootwork has an animistic foundation. Animistic philosophy addresses each element or aspect of nature as being alive. Objects from nature are imbued with animism and ashe, so they have a universal energy force within them that connects us all like an umbilical cord. To simply use herbs, flowers, stones, bones, fire, or water without paying homage to their life force insults spirit. In Haiti, for example, spirits are believed to "mount" humans, helping them to carry out healing work. Healers under the influence of various lwa (spirits) will fall into a trancelike state; some dance during healings while others sing or chant. In the United States, many healers in the African American community commence their work with prayers, psalms, or song. Bringing together spirit with healing work is an exciting experience and it is also a distinctive aspect of herbalism inspired by ATRs (African Traditional Religions). To summarize, yes there are tools, equipment, and methods, but there is also spirit, the spirit of nature, the ancestor spirits, and the spirit within yourself. Be sure to remain attentive to your intuition as you work roots because often it is the way spirit communicates and assists with healing work.

CHAPTER THREE

You Reap What You Sow

Planting with Spirit/Harvesting Ashe

Planting: The Magical and Physical Seed

While writing this book, I could not help thinking about my parents. They have passed on, but they are alive in my memory as creative muses. Though their parents have connections to the South, both of my parents were raised in the North. For reasons unbeknownst to me, they decided as a young couple not to repeat that experience and give their own children a different upbringing. They moved us to the country and although we hated it at first, I realize it has made me who I am. My childhood experiences have inspired my painting, poetry, and writing. In large part it is those experiences in my youth that are the impetus for this herbal guide.

My mother and father seemed to adapt to country living almost too easily. We quickly went from renting a small cottage by the lake to living off the land for nearly two years as my father built our home from the ground up. Before I knew it, Dad was hunting deer, fishing, and gardening, not just for fun but also as the mainstay of our sustenance. We supplemented this with buying milk, eggs, and a half side of beef and similar foods from local farmers who were also my parents' friends. The gardening is something my father did until shortly before his death. The same holds true for my mother. She had an incredible green thumb and could take tomato plants from seed to flower to fruit indoors, off-season—without the assistance of grow lights, mind you.

When you are a teenager the most important thing seems to be fitting in and being cool. I found my parents' homespun ways more than a little embarrassing. During the period when our house was being built, we lived in a log cabin with a fireplace and kerosene stove as the only sources of heat. We had no running water for nearly two years. This meant that we had to do a lot of physical work to accomplish ordinary tasks that most people take for granted. Like it or not, we had a window into the daily lives of those who had lived well before us as we walked in their shoes in some respects. I credit this with cultivating creativity and helping me understand how to live in accordance with nature.

Between my parents and our grandfather, who was born on a slave plantation in 1890, I learned how to make organic fertilizer from ordinary kitchen refuse and from cast-offs from fresh lake fish, the right times for planting, how to harvest various fruits and vegetables, and then to preserve the harvest by freezing and canning. I even learned how to make fruit wine and moonshine, should push come to shove.

Since in many ways this book is a tribute to the ancestors and to those who have lived close to the land, part of its lesson is to encourage you to learn from your parents—even though it may seem "uncool"—from their parents if they are still around, and from the elders in your community. Appreciate cultural heritage, but also bring your own energy into traditions to help keep them alive and.

Growing one's food from seed to flower to fruit is one of life's more satisfying activities. The move I spoke of occurred when I was about seven. We moved from a stone's throw away from Manhattan to a place in rural New Jersey that is called the Delaware Valley, two hundred miles away. I grew up in Jersey tomato, blueberry, and eggplant-growing country. Our school bus ride took us past numerous fields of various types of grain, sheep, horses, and cows. In fact, the county over from ours, Cumberland County, is one of the country's largest producers of eggplant. This was not idyllic in the least; there were practical and social difficulties. As African Americans, we were an extreme minority. This, in the long run, allowed me to have more time to commune with nature, observe my surroundings, and connect with my people when the opportunity presented itself.

Whatever we planted seemed to bear fruit in southern New Jersey—it is no wonder why it is called the Garden State. I have many memories of planting, growing, and of the harvesting season, and here is one that paints a portrait of that time.

Around 6:30 a.m., the foggy mist skips daintily over the silky green lake as we head over the dirt hill to Aunt Edith's place. Aunt Edith's house is freshly painted; the cinder blocks are now turquoise. Her yard dwarfs the bungalow tucked beneath sweeping mimosa trees with their fringed pink and white delicately scented blooms. We plant things on her land—she has areas of land without trees, a rarity in our wet and wooded neighborhood.

Aunt Edith's favorite plants are pole limas. The bean in my hand mimics the yin-yang symbol, but in a dull dry skin and creamy grayish tan color. We start tillin' and weedin' before it gets too hot, but when it does, the old folk drink beer and give me a swig, too, which goes nicely with our salted Jersey tomatoes.

On weekends we wake even earlier to go to the larger fields used by various companies. We live near the lands farmed by Green Giant, Hunt's, and other commercial produce companies. After the workings of their huge machines, so much is left behind to harvest. We go in and pick and pick and pick some more, till I think or hope I have cramps in my hands—bushels and bushels of beans. We are careful in case anyone official might see us and put a stop to our work, but fortunately, they never do.

When we arrive at home, Ma has picnic tables set out in the front yard, to make our work easier. It is time to put up (preserve) the harvest to see us through fall, winter, and into the spring. Thwack! The bushels of beans hit the table hard. We begin our sorting and snapping of the string beans—this consumes the better half of the day. Then the next day, we put the beans "up" for winter.

In suburbia I hold my bean, remembering as I stroke it. It is a perfect teleport into my youth. Beginning to the left, and ending not quite right—the pod where egg and seed meet. Snap one; snap two; three and four. "Mommy, were you listening to me at all?" my daughter asks impatiently. Spread the soil and plant your seeds, girl . . . I dream on.

The water boils, and I let the snapped beans tumble free from their cobalt blue Tupperware colander. Minced onions and garlic sizzle in the seasoned cast iron skillet as I sprinkle on some dried cayenne, pepper, and coarse sea salt. A splash of apple vinegar followed by the cubed potatoes—plop, splash, on top of the green beans.

Today, even though I live in an urban suburb in Illinois, I am lucky to live on land with black, humus-rich soil, which we have enhanced with our own kitchen compost. The rich soil enables me to remain in touch with the Earth Mother through gardening; though my patch of earth is now small, it is still my own. On my land I continue to plant magical and literal seeds—hopes and dreams for the future as well as tributes to my people.

Living far away from the home of my family, paying these tributes is something that came to me intuitively. I recalled how many families had cemetery plots on their land. Being hundreds of miles away, it made sense to try to pay some sort of visual homage to my departed loved ones on my land. Richard Westmacott wrote one of the most in-depth books on the African American ways of gardening and maintaining yards, *African-American Gardens and Yards in the Rural South*.[1] Westmacott highlights ways of gardening, tending land, and maintaining a yard that is distinctively African American. These include having transplanted plants from nearby forests such as dogwood trees, which is something my family did. My parents also transplanted mountain laurel, which grew profusely in the area. Planting memorial plants to pay tribute to someone you love that has departed this earth is another specific aspect of Black Southern gardens. The inclusion of symbolic magical talismans like seashells, coins, or other special objects as part of the garden décor is another feature. Utilization of rocks, particularly river rocks, alongside the pathway and bottles hung in trees as protective amulets is also common. Robert Farris Thompson discusses the bottle tree phenomenon in *Flash of the Spirit*, along with the other ways people in the African diaspora go about imbuing their gardens with spirit.

Thompson also notes that in Southern tradition, landowners often buried their deceased family members on the property,[2] as I had also observed. This changes the character of the yard, making it part cemetery and part garden—bringing life and death together. Here is the story of an actual garden I planted. Perhaps it will give you ideas for making your own spirit garden as a protective amulet to your home and a tribute to your ancestors:

The Pathway Home

We are ambling down the path, boxes and bags held snug, when the vision of a new home in the distance offsets my balance.

I pause. A cursory glance over the barren gray dirt that someone thought was a yard and a plan hatches: a couple of forsythia bushes over there; a smatter of deep purple Dutch iris here; maybe some double-blooming, raspberry-scented peonies right there; a cluster of sweetly fragrant lilies closest to the front door. Ah, that would be a nice touch. At long last—a creative plan to fill the void.

We waddle back and forth, arms brimming with precious possessions. Just before dusk with boxes, bags, paintings, sculptures, and tatty furniture tucked safely indoors, it is time to venture back outside. After living in the inner city with barely a tree over five years old, having a yard, however barren and small, is emancipation.

What would Mama think?

There is none of the bucolic splendor here that I grew up with. This tight and tidy brick two-flat is only a stone's throw away from the L tracks.

Once, the view from my bedroom window was of a verdant lake rimmed with sweeping pines and sleepy willows. Now I look out over the canyon created by the expressway and a river of ever-flowing, noisy vehicles.

As an artist, I realize the world is as beautiful as imagination permits.

I plow the soil diligently with my hand tools, flipping her over and over again with my pitchfork. Soon enough it becomes evident that, like me, she is still very fertile. As I dig down deep, I find the soil to be as rich and black as a Yoruban queen. Within these dark depths, I plant an array of seeds and bulbs:

Lullabies at night for the little one.

Sunny daffodils by day to light the way for the boys.

Purple pansies, Mama's color and flower in her memory.

Hope, for the healthy birth of the little girl growing within my still-flat belly. Sunflowers, narcissi, and a variety of botanical tulips for my grandmothers. Negro spirituals, as a tribute to Grandpop.

Shiny pennies are tossed for luck.

Yarrow for my ultra-strong Great-grandma Louise.

Sensual Bourbonnais roses for my dear Aunt Rose.

Daily water and fire rituals for clarity, strength, and protection.

Columbine Spring Song for my second mum, Iris, who radiates gentility, power, and grace.

Rites of fertility, recipes for continued health, creativity, and the infinite capacity to love.

These are anchored by a round cairn of stone symbolic of my soul mate.

All set behind a white-washed picket fence that seemed to begin aging as soon as it was erected (sprinkled with goofer dust to bar evil spirits from entry) . . . and so it went for over a decade.

The little one and I head up the path. Projects, chores, responsibilities, appointments, obligations, that heady scent of lilac, Bourbonnais roses, and the remaining narcissi muddle my thoughts. The path from home is not the straight walk it once was.

Today my path is strewn with leaves, stems, flowers, and looming shadows.

Veronica Speedwell leans over each side of the walkway gossiping with the little chrysanthemums. The peonies now need their own zip code, but at least the lilies keep to themselves. The black-eyed Susans are spreading everywhere, but the cronewort, *Artemisia vulgaris* (where the hell did she come from?), thankfully is just as thick as she is tall. I hear her cackle coming and going, though sometimes it is just barely audible. She and her feathery leaves look like helping hands. Tough sage green on top, tender, soft, and silver beneath, tassels above all, lending sultry airs all around.

Mysteriously, cronewort has taken up residence outside our front door. Where once there was order, plans, and direction to my garden, there is now a lush green space, whose semblance of order lies beneath, at the base of the garden, within the roots.

Buried remnants of well-laid plans intermingle with seashells and pennies from days of old. My garden is now a sanctuary. Birds, bees, children, and weary commuters find soul food and solace as they make their way through the world.

This place people used to call a yard is now more of a Healer's Thatch. Approaching a wildflower prairie, this space is sheltered by a teeming forest of sunflowers with the cronewort and her stylish tresses acting as gatekeeper.

I could go on and on about my tangled mass of stems, overgrown perennials, strangling weeds, and stinging thistles. Most often, though, I just want to get home and latch that decrepit gate behind me.

No matter that as of this spring, the elder boy towers over me and I feel the rustling of Oya's skirts as he passes in pursuit of hopes and dreams beyond my reach. Though they are gangly and a bit unruly, still, I know that as each child grows, the sunflowers will present their aspirations to the sun.

Our toddler and the newly transplanted French lavender, rose scented geranium, geranium chamomile, and hyssop vie for the warming rays of the sun and merciful light along with a precious bit of space to call their own.

Stooping over to lessen the load, the reflection in the puddle reveals a wide-hipped, thick-legged Black woman, flecks of gray intermingled in her reddish brown Afro.

She looks back at me with the fixed gaze of one-who-sees.

Time to stop overlooking the ancient wisdom that has taken root at my doorstep. Tonight I will cut some cronewort for the first time. I'll rub her between my palms, inhale her camphorlike aroma deeply, and then place a bit of her green blood on my third eye to enhance my foresight. Next, I'll stuff the stems and leaves in a jar and drench them in safflower oil.

While I'm waiting for the Crone to release her powers into the oil, I'll do another cutting. This bunch of the feathered Hag will be braided, tied with hemp string, and once dried, she will be lit. The flames will be snuffed, so only her husky voice remains, to be waved over the doorstep that she faces and protects.

"Cronewort, bless this path, stoop, and entry and all those who cross this way," I implore in hushed tones by the light of the full moon. Once the moon completes her full cycle, I'll strain a bit of that precious green oil and pour it on my naked body, letting it penetrate my tired soul, aching joints, and Earth-shaped belly. When I am healed, I'll work on my soul mate, my children, and perhaps others in need of her life juice.

Time to use what has been given and to realize that I am no longer a slender girl eagerly searching for homes on distant shores.

Woman of the house.

Planter of seeds.

Tiller of dreams.

Too old to call maiden and too young to call crone.

THE SACRED GARDEN

This is an introduction to an idea that is a spiritually reward-ing way of gardening in the astral or spiritual dimension. My friend and fellow author Connie Rodriguez wrote this excerpt and it is drawn from her book *Sacred Codes: Ancient Keys for Unlocking Soul Awareness.*[3]

"I often use a sacred garden in imagery as a starting point to journey to another time, to the cosmic realm, or to meet a power animal which then takes me to one of the spiritual realms. My sacred garden has become the portal into these realms. You can actually find this sacred garden in my yard in the physical world, but it is also where I go to in my inner world to journey to the mystical realms. It has become one of my most favorite stable attractor sites.

"This imaginal sacred garden shifts and changes with my inner needs. It has a beautiful goldfish and koi pond with a waterfall as its central feature.

"It has a wonderful turtle that is sometimes sunning himself on one of the rocks around the pond. It also has colorful flow-ers, cymbidium orchids, and ferns that shimmer next to the pond. Surrounding the pond are a few Gold Coast pines that give a shel-tered feeling in my garden. To the left of the pond is a large flat rock, one that I can lay on to sunbathe or to go to other places. I also have an imaginal upright stone that anchors the garden and has become an altar where I place gifts I have received from my inner travels. At the base of this stone is a beautiful crystal and nautilus shell that I was recently given on one excursion in the imaginal realm. Just beyond this standing stone is an arbor cov-ered with red roses. When I walk through this arbor I can often walk down to a sandy beach where I meet with my inner advisors as taught by my professor. Sometimes I will bring a problem or concern to them and we will sit on the sand in a circle while I am advised of what I may need to think about."

–Constance Rodriguez, PhD, Depth Therapist and Intuitive Counselor

Creating a Spirit Garden

No one can tell you how to make your own spirit garden because all of the seeds for it are planted within your soul. I can make a few suggestions for your consideration as you plan such a garden.

› First and foremost, you need to allow yourself plenty of rest, and still time. Still time is the time you set aside where you are not concerned about work, sustenance, your love life, family, or anything. It is simply when you can be quiet and exist, observing what thoughts occur once your slate of concerns has been wiped clean. Allow yourself still time and meditation so that you can tap into your intuition—your spirit within.

› Having a blank book in whatever pattern or style will inspire you to record recollections, dreams, and thoughts about your garden. Keep this and a pen handy, tucked away in a place that is easily accessible so that you can use it as the thoughts arise.

› If this is to pay tribute or remind you of someone you love who has passed on, try to think about the things, colors, sounds, textures, flowers, vegetables, fruits, and herbs that person or animal enjoyed. Write these down in your spirit garden journal. Make plans to purchase seeds or borrow cuttings from a neighbor during planting season.

› Consider the zodiac—this was a huge pastime with our ancestors in the United States. Do you want to arrange a bed of flowers or herbs in the shape of your, another person's, or an animal's astrological sign? Consider the strengths and weaknesses of each sign.

› An alternative in line with the zodiac would be to plant your garden using hex patterns (popular with African American followers of Pow Wow[4]). You could also work with a powerful African amulet like the ankh, a symbol of everlasting life.

› Rather than plant in a pattern, you could simply mark out the pattern of the astrological sign, hex sign, or African amulet using stones.

› Collect textured materials to put in the garden. Consider sea glass (glass smoothed by the ocean so it has no rough edges), patterned marbles, pieces of flat rounded glass (these are sold at garden centers and craft stores for indoor gardening and candle environments), charged quartz crystal, river rocks, or driftwood.

Points to Remember

1. Quartz crystal makes your garden area conducive to vision quests, divination, and healing energy.

2. River rocks invoke the spirit of Oshun, orisha of sensuality, beauty, and sexuality.

3. Driftwood invokes the spirit of Yemaya-Ologun, mother orisha who nurtures and protects her children.

› Consider statuary—some people like to put saints, the Virgin Mary, or the Virgin of Guadeloupe in their gardens. Others prefer earth goddesses from ancient Egypt like the Triple Goddess symbol, Goddess of the Nile, or even a bust of Nefertiti. Still others have patrons whose energy they like to keep nearby. These include many different types of Buddhas, Saint Francis, Santa Barbara, Black Madonnas, Kwan Yin (goddess of compassion), and Laksmi (goddess of prosperity, sensuality and abundance).

› Borrowing from the Cayman Islanders and Southern African Americans, you could also try keeping a swept yard. This bears some resemblance in spirit to Japanese sand gardens. Cayman Islanders are known for drawing out wave patterns that can be seen in the moonlight. African Americans sweep these types of gardens smooth with a brushwood broom. You could use your magical besom. The garden must be kept free of foot tracks and weeds; it is a labor of love. These types of garden are still seen in parts of West Africa.[5] An area devoted to the swept yard will be especially appealing to those who enjoy a place of quiet contemplation but who may lack the green thumb for growing plants. A swept yard is covered in soil or you can bring in white sand and each week you sweep the yard (or even a small area of the yard) into subtle patterns to instill a feeling of inner peace.

> Finally, a great deal can be said by the selection of the plants themselves. Plants featured in the following chapters that were brought to the Americas and Caribbean by enslaved Africans include watermelon, okra, black-eyed peas, sesame, eggplant, yams, peanut, cantaloupe, and West Indian gherkin.[6] You can also use plants to symbolically suggest a person as I have done in my spirit garden.

There are infinite ways to create an African spirit garden. The main limitations are set by your imagination so stay in touch with your intuition, angels, or muses, listen intently and start with small, manageable increments that are easy to complete.

Creative Gathering

Some people become really intimidated by the idea of gardening, figuring they don't have enough land or any land of their own to plant in and till. For folk living in cities, apartments, and other tight spaces where land comes at a premium price, the primary source for gathering of herbs may well be specialty catalogs, health food stores, and online.

Even within this commercial arena the way you go about gathering is critical, and the relationships developed can be meaningful, educational, and fun. Things to look for are:

> Are the herbs ethically harvested? Be careful about barks and roots; some herbs like echinacea are overharvested and face extinction.

> Are the herbs organically grown? This is the safest method for personal care products and consumables.

> Are the prices fair, without excessive markups? Do some research and price comparisons.

> Are the herbs usually in stock, available without delays?

> Is the source convenient and practical for you?

> Is a knowledgeable person available to answer your questions?

> Start out with a local shop if possible, but as you become comfortable with creating your own brews, branch out into wholesale. Buying herbs in bulk saves big bucks!

Other Suggestions to City Dwellers

> Look for freshness (bright color, no mold or mildew, strong scent) and expiration dates on herbs.

> Grow your favorite herbs in pots on the windowsill, terrace, or inside using grow lights.

> Visit your local farmers market, investigate organic whole food co-ops, or drive outside the city to support roadside farm stands.

A Note about Wildcrafting

If you are fortunate enough to go wildcrafting (gathering fresh herbs from the forest, fields, or other locales), or if you have a garden of your own, here is a ritual to ensure a good harvest. Make sure you have permission and are not harvesting on restricted land or taking fragile or "at-risk" plants when wildcrafting. Here is a working list of such plants archived by United Plant Savers.[7] You will want to use these with a great deal of discernment if you are dealing with wholesalers or buying in quantity as well:

Partial List of At-Risk Plants

American Ginseng *(Panax quinquefolius)*

Black Cohosh *(Actaea racemosa, Cimicifuga racemosa)*

Bloodroot *(Sanguinaria canadensis)*

Blue Cohosh *(Caulophyllum thalictroides)*

Echinacea *(Echinacea* sp.*)*

Eyebright *(Euphrasia* sp.*)*

Goldenseal *(Hydrastis canadensis)*

Lady's Slipper Orchid *(Cypripedium* sp.*)*

Lomatium *(Lomatium dissectum)*

Osha *(Ligusticum porteri, L.* sp.*)*

Peyote *(Lophophora williamsii)*

Slippery Elm *(Ulmus rubra)*

Sundew *(Drosera* sp.*)*

Trillium, Beth Root *(Trillium* sp.*)*

True Unicorn (*Aletris farinosa)*

Venus' Fly Trap *(Dionaea muscipula)*

Virginia Snakeroot *(Aristolochia serpentaria)*

Wild Yam *(Dioscorea villosa, D.* sp.*)*

Some "To Watch" Plants

Arnica (*Arnica* sp.)

Butterfly Weed (*Asclepias tuberosa*)

Cascara Sagrada (*Rhamnus purshimia*)

Chaparro (*Castela emoryi*)

Elephant Tree (*Bursera microphylla*)

Gentian (*Gentiana* sp.)

Goldthread (*Coptis* sp.)

Kava (*Piper methysticum*) (Hawaii only)

Lobelia (*Lobelia* sp.)

Maidenhair Fern (*Adiantum pedatum*)

Mayapple (*Podophyllum peltatum*)

Oregon Grape (*Mahonia* sp.)

Partridge Berry (*Mitchella repens*)

Pink Root (*Spigelia marilandica*)

Pipsissewa (*Chimaphila umbellata*)

Stone Root (*Collinsonia canadensis*)

Stream Orchid (*Epipactis gigantea*)

White Sage (*Salvia apiana*)

Wild Indigo (*Baptisia tinctoria*)

Yerba Mansa (*Anemopsis californica*)

Ancestor Harvest Offering

Before harvest, it is important to make offerings to the ancestor in the earth, thanking her for her fertility. Here is an offering to try:

Bring fresh fruit and vegetables of the season, a white candle, and matches to a fresh water source (pond, river, stream, lake) closest to you. Those without a body of water can still pay tribute using a portable fountain. Set out fruit special to your family or heritage. Clear a space, down to the dirt, for the pillar candle. Light. Begin your prayer of thanks. "I know that you were here in my beginning and that you will be here in the end. Blessed Be. Thank you for always being with me, for influencing, shaping and making me whole. Blessed Be. I lay these fruits out for you to partake in the presence of our elixirs of life. Blessed Be. I am yours, you are mine, in body, mind, and spirit. Blessed Be." Bow your head. Listen to the ancestor's response. When you are ready, extinguish the candle and take it with you, but leave the fruit out as food for the ancestors at the site.

PLANTING AND HARVESTING FOLKLORE

The book *Folklore of Adams County, Illinois* (Dr. Harry Middleton Hyatt, Folklore of Adams County, Illinois: Memoirs of the Alma Egan Hyatt Foundation (New York: The E. Cabella-French Printing and Publishing Corporation, 1935)) is a wellspring of Negro folklore and that of immigrants from Germany, Ireland, Wales, and other places in Europe. Here is a confluence of superstitions from that book concerning planting and harvesting:

Plant seeds as soon as the soil has been prepared or you will not be successful with them.

Rusty nails or old iron placed around plants helps them grow better. This is likely "Negro" folklore because the idea of using rusty nails is prevalent in African American Hoodoo and is traced back to the magical attributes given to metallurgy and metalsmiths, which is shared in depth in my previous book, *Sticks, Stones, Roots and Bones: Hoodoo, Mojo and Conjuring with Herbs* (St. Paul: Llewellyn, 2004).

Everything planted by a pregnant woman grows well; nothing planted by a menstruating woman grows. This is sympathetic magic; a pregnant woman is fertile, with life growing inside her, thus what she touches will also grow, whereas a menstruating woman is not pregnant and might not be fertile so the opposite outcome is predicted.

Root crops should be planted during the moonlight in the shape of the lower part of the body.

Plant seeds when the moon is full and they will grow well.

The sign of Cancer is moist so planting during that sign brings great success to the crops. Astrology plays a very prominent role in African American culture. A great deal of the planting guidance centers around mimicking shapes of the astrological signs.

Seeds that grow above ground should be planted only in the morning.

Underground (root) crops should be planted in the afternoon.

Most seeds planted at high noon will grow well.

Sowing seeds on Good Friday is lucky.

Mash eggshells and let them stand in water. Pour off the liquid. It will help flowers blossom. This is the type of simple fertilizer my mother made. She also used coffee grind fertilizer.

Transplant flowers by moonlight for successful growth.

Harvesting Leaves

Look for leaves of a consistent green color without brown or yellow spots. Harvest mid-morning, after the dew has evaporated. Gather leaves before the plant begins to flower. For plants such as basil or oregano that have long growing seasons, pinch back tops to prevent flowering. (Flowering takes energy away from the main body of the plant.) Keep herbs separated by type, and tie the stems loosely together in a bundle with twine or hemp string. Until you are very familiar with all of the herbs, it is best to label the bundles and date them as well. Hang them up to dry immediately after harvesting to prevent mildew or deterioration.

Hang herb bundles stem-up in an area with good circulation, away from direct sunlight. The ideal temperature for the first twenty-four hours is 90 degrees, followed by 75–80 degrees the rest of the time. Most herbal bundles will dry within two to three weeks. Petals and leaves should feel light, crisp, and paper-like. If there are small buds or tiny leaves, which may fall off during the drying time, create a roomy muslin bag to encase flowers and leaves, and tie them loosely with twine or hemp string at the stems. This is particularly important with seed-dropping plants such as fennel or sunflowers. When the herbs are completely dry, store the whole leaf and stem away from direct sunlight in dark glass or stainless steel airtight containers.

Harvesting Flowers

Select healthy flowers in the early afternoon during dry weather conditions. Flowers are extremely delicate. Take extra care not to bruise the petals—refrain from touching them, and cut from the stem, allowing the flowers to drop into a basket. Dry smaller, more delicate flowers such as lavender and chamomile whole; hang them upside down, tied with twine over a muslin cloth or large bowl, or wrap them loosely with muslin to retain dried buds.

Use fresh flowers whenever possible. You may also freeze them in an ice cube tray filled with spring water.

Harvesting Seeds

Collect seeds on a warm, dry day. Seeds need to dry in a warm, airy environment. Make provisions to catch the quickly drying seeds by placing a bowl or box underneath the hanging plants.

Harvesting Bark

Bark peels easiest on damp days. Choose a young tree or bush—if possible one that has already been pruned, cut, or taken down naturally by wind or stormy conditions to prevent damage or even death to the plant. Stripping too much bark from a tree will kill it. A thoughtful approach to Mother Nature's gifts is essential. Bark may harbor insects or moss, so wash it first and allow it to dry flat on waxed paper in a location that is well ventilated and away from direct sunlight.

Harvesting Roots

Roots are ready for collecting after autumn harvest. Dig up roots after their plant has begun to wither and die. Extract the whole root while trying not to bruise it. Like bark, roots need to be cleaned before they are dried. They also require ethical harvesting to yield ashe. Cut roots into small sections and dry them in an oven set between 120 to 140 degrees. Turn and check regularly. Roots should feel light and airy like sawdust when fully dried. For marshmallow root, peel away the top layer of skin before drying in this manner.

Harvesting Berries

Use the same procedure as for bark, but remember that berries and fruits take a long time to dry, about twice as long as leaves. You will know when they are fully dry because they will become very light, wrinkled, and reduced in size by nearly half. Turn frequently and check for leaking juices. Replace paper below them often to prevent the growth of bacteria or mold.

Winter

CHAPTER FOUR

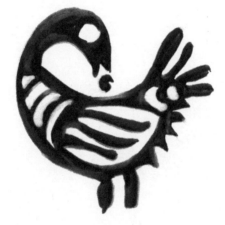

Winter by the Fire

A Season of Love, Remembrance, Dreaming, and the Elder

Multicultural Winter Holidays

We begin each year during winter, a time in temperate zones when many outward signs of life are dormant. This is the time after harvest. A time when we bond together indoors, enjoying the abundance of the harvest season's fruits and vegetables, as friends, lovers, and family. Yule (also called winter solstice), Chanukah, Christmas, Kwanzaa, New Year, and Saint Valentine's Day are holidays that reinforce our desire for togetherness. The chill in the air and the dramatically reduced presence of the sun play into our need to pull inside. We pull into ourselves as readily as we pull into our homes. This is a time to balance introspection with finding clever ways of demonstrating our feelings for others.

Winter is also a time to plan and to dream, as it is the season of the sleeping bear, and the time of mid-winter dreaming festivals for some Native American nations. The elder, symbol of the winter season of life, is also celebrated. Yes, it is a challenging time, but if it is approached with an appreciation for what it offers us, it can be a free gift to all. Why not light your favorite candle or some incense as you tuck into this chapter exploring a variety of ways to enhance health during winter?

Yule and Winter Solstice

Living with Candlelight:
Illuminating the Mind, Body, and Spirit

As winter approaches and the amount of daily sunlight dwindles, many of us crave more hours of light. Since our earliest days, we as humans have snuggled close to the fireside for comfort, warmth, fellowship, nourishment, and the light that fire generates. Naturally then, those of us maintaining a natural home tend fires of various sizes and shapes, including the hearth, stove, fireplace, chimenea, barbeque pit, as well as incense and candles.

Candles are one of the more appealing forms of fire for many reasons. They are utilized to set a mood and give off fragrance. Candles are used as the focal point of celebrations, vigils, feasts, and special meals. They are portable and accessible to just about everyone. Candles are also inexpensive compared to some of the other options such as installing a wood-burning stove. This section is designed to assist those interested in holistic health to select and utilize candles in a wholesome, life-affirming, seasonal way.

Aromatherapy and Aromacology

Scent is one of the more alluring qualities of candles. There have been many books that explore scent in relation to holistic health—a few of my favorites are listed in the bibliography. While there have been no definitive, large-scaled, scientific studies pointing out the specific benefits of aromatherapy, it has a time-honored tradition in holistic health.

Aromatherapy is a term coined by a French chemist named Rene-Maurice Gattefosse in the early 20th century. He is believed to have burned himself and grabbed the nearest thing to him, which happened to be lavender oil. He noticed his burn healed quickly, and he launched a full-scale study of the benefits of aromatic botanicals in healing. This field of healing with aromatic botanicals is called aromatherapy.

Aromatherapy is a technique that calls for aromatic plant substances to be released. Typically this is done through water (baths or hydrosols), oil (like essential oils), or fire (incense, candles, and aromatic wood like mesquite or aloeswood). Aromatherapy is used for a variety of physical complaints, symptoms, and conditions including menopause, insomnia, pain, swelling, PMS, burns, wounds, colds, and influenza.

Aromacology is a newer term, which focuses more on the mind/spirit connection between aroma, a positive mood, and health. Aromacology utilizes aromatic botanicals to alleviate mental or spiritual discomforts. These discomforts and diseases include agitation, nervousness, listlessness, tension, sorrow, anger, mourning, addictions, and anxiety.

While aromatherapy and aromacology have become industry buzzwords to generate sales for fragrant products, there are professional practitioners of this healing technique called aromatherapists. Some aromatherapists are registered, certified professionals who are licensed to practice in certain countries. When considering aromatherapeutic or aromacology applications of aromatics for the home, such as candles, it is best to conduct independent research if you have the resources, or consult with a professional aromatherapist rather than depend on product advertisements. The NAHA (National Association for Holistic Aromatherapy) is a good source, online at *naha.org*. They provide a list of national and international registered aromatherapists.

Scented Candles

Essential oils are primary tools of the aromatherapist. As the name implies, an essential oil is the condensed essence of a plant. Plant parts used to produce essential oils are the medicinal parts of the plant, typically the berry, root, leaf, stem, bark, or flower. Essential oils are taken in a variety of ways, dispensed topically, and vaporized. When enjoying candles that have been scented naturally, you are experiencing vaporized essential oils or another concentrated plant substance called an absolute.

Absolutes are sometimes referred to as natural fragrances. Absolutes are very expensive, as the process for creating them involves extracting scent from plants whose fragrances are difficult to capture and condense. The absolutes you might find in the very finest candles are rose, nag champa, hyacinth, neroli, or lilac. Many people concerned with holistic health will seek out candles scented with pure essential oils and absolutes because they are nature-based substances.

Fragrance oils are called by many different names: synthetic, nature identical oils (NIOs), or simply oils. People who suffer from airborne allergies seem to have a particularly tough time with synthetic fragrance oils. They make most people in my home who are sensitive to artificial scents sneeze. Tenders of the natural home may find a synthetic scent to be offensive and out of place within their home, however closely it approximates a natural scent. Often fragrance oils are strong-smelling and lack the subtlety of essential oils from plants.

Moreover, there is a group of carcinogens suspected to exist within the synthetic fragrance oils sometimes used in candle manufacture. These are called phthalates. Phthalates are chemicals used to dilute fragrances, making them more soluble in the wax. They are also linked to respiratory problems.

People who argue in favor of fragrance oils are quick to point out that natural does not necessarily mean healthy. There is a suggestion that fragrance oils burn better than essential oils, but this is unfounded. We do realize there are poison plants that are as natural as they are deadly. There are also known allergens in the natural plant world, including some of the conifers (pine especially), as well as cinnamon bark oil and clove bud oil.

Holistic health advocates and manufacturers who also fit into this group feel one of the best features of essential oils and absolutes is the source of the scent. Knowing the true source is valuable to many people, and you will notice it is a recurring theme in this section. Knowing the source of the scent makes it easy to learn the botanical's tradition in healing, its magical symbolism, and its spiritual connotations.

There is no definitive study to support one type of oil over another. Spiritually, there is no question. Pure essential oils have a venerable past and a tradition of healing in numerous cultures. For many people, ancient oils like sandalwood, frankincense, myrrh, or the celebrated lavender that sparked aromatherapy, cannot be replaced by synthetics.

CANDLE HISTORY

Thousands of years before Gattefosse, fragrant botanicals were used in ancient North Africa, including Egypt, where candlesticks were found dated to 1600 BCE.

Fragrant oils enjoyed use in the early cultures of India, Persia, and the Mediterranean.

The Romans made candles with wicks and wax much like ours. The wicks were made from rolled papyrus and treated with seawater to slow the burning rate.

Pliny the Younger reported on candles made from tallow in 1st-century Avignon, France.

Emperor Constantine used candles in the Christian church, for Easter services in the 4th century.

Candlemas, February 2, is a special holiday with a venerable history. Candlemas is the day of blessing and distributing candles for places of worship and the home.

THE WHOLE BALL OF WAX

These days we have choices in so many elements of our lives that were once unthinkable. This is true for candles as well as just about every other product on the market. Here is a brief summary of the more common types of materials candle wax is made from and the pros and cons of each.

Beeswax—comes from bees. Beeswax candles are long burning, sweet smelling, natural, and aromatic. Beeswax candles are considered a good value and an important contribution to the natural home because they come from an almost entirely natural source, apart from their formation. You can purchase these from craftsmen and beekeepers at farmers' markets in your community. The con against beeswax candles is that their price is generally higher than other candles. Vegans and followers of some religions would not find an insect product like beeswax to be in keeping with their beliefs.

Paraffin—the most common candle material today. Paraffin is a petroleum by-product. Paraffin wax candles are easy to find, burn efficiently, and are inexpensive to purchase. The problem many people find with paraffin wax is that it is derived from a fossil fuel (coal), which is not renewable or earth-friendly. Because of its source, some users find that paraffin wax candles give off more soot and leave an unpleasant after-smell in the room. As a compromise, some manufacturers are using food-grade paraffin wax to make what they call healthier candles.

Soy–candles are said to burn efficiently, cleanly, and to hold fragrance very well. American farmers grow soybeans, and by purchasing soy candles you help support their efforts. Purchasing in this manner means a lot to those involved with right-living. Soy is natural but not derived from animals, making it accept-able for vegans. It is also a renewable source, growing in abundance domestically. On the downside, soy candles may not be available in every area, and they sometimes cost more than paraffin wax candles because their current demand is lower.

Which Wick Is Which

Every element of the candle and how it is burned is worthy of careful consideration by keepers of the natural home. The wick has drawn a great deal of attention because consumers in the early 1970s discovered that some contain lead or lead alloys. Candles containing any lead at all can release up to twenty percent of that metal into the air. Children under the age of six are most affected by lead—lead poisoning can cause damage to the nervous system and the brain. Government tests found burning a candle with a lead wick for just fifteen to thirty days could raise a child's lead level.[1]

Some candles, particularly those from China, still contain metal-lic substances within the wick. The alloy-containing wicks are a bit trickier to avoid, and it is likely that more of them exist on the market sold as tin/zinc wicks. This is good reason to consider the source from which you purchase your candles or candle making supplies; reputable sources participating in the ban and labeling their products' contents are recommended.

The National Candle Association (NCA) recommends testing candles that have never been burned at the store before purchasing them if you are suspicious about their contents. To test for lead, rub a piece of clean white paper across the wick. If there remains a trace of a metallic, grayish color on the paper, the particular candle uses lead or a metal alloy within the wick.

Never leave candles unattended, and be sure to snuff candles before leaving the home. We seek enlightenment and tend to spend more time in winter—more than any other season—near fire, in the form of candlelight, smoldering incense, the kitchen stove, or an actual fireside. Here is an aromatic way to incorporate the element of fire:

Yule Fire and Ice Reflection Ritual

Here is a fun way to gather the family in a simply beautiful Yule project and ritual. With supervision, most children can easily make this themselves; it makes a fun family project.

1. Gather your favorite evergreens. Choose a few cuttings each from such winter favorites as holly with berries, juniper with berries, cedar, spruce, or pine needles. If available, add a few tiny birch pinecones as well (these are one inch or less).

2. Pour water into a three-inch deep rectangular plastic (flexible) container, half full. Place three to six naturally scented beeswax, soy, or essential oil scented candles into the container. The candles should be four inches tall and three to four inches wide.

3. Add the evergreens and berries to the container in a pleasing arrangement around the candles. Cover the greens with more water so they'll appear to float once frozen. Be careful not to over-fill; the plastic container should be two-thirds full of water in the end.

4. Place in the freezer until frozen (or outdoors if it's cold enough). Freeze until solid.

5. Slide out the rectangular ice block with the evergreens and candles frozen inside. Turn onto a fire-proof plate (a high-fired glazed ceramic plate would serve well) or an old cookie sheet covered with foil. You can accentuate the display by placing polished stones (black, white, or natural river rocks) or polished glass beads (clear, sparkle, blue, or black) around the edges of the ice.

6. Light the candles. Say a winter prayer, offer a blessing, and be thankful to our essential elements of fire, water, air, and earth.

CANDLE SAFETY TIPS

Always trim the candle and remove matches, trimming, wrapping or other debris before lighting. Candlewick should be trimmed at least ¼ inch before lighting.

Use a proper candleholder for the candle type. Make sure it is fireproof.

Burn candles away from drafts, vents, fans, or hallways to avoid setting clothing on fire. Do not burn candles where children are playing. Place candles away from dried flowers, magazines, drapery, or other flammable materials.

Burn candles one hour per inch in diameter. For example, a candle that is three inches wide should be burned for three hours. After burning, once the candle wax pools have solidified but the candle is still warm, gently rub the candle upward to reshape it. This is called candle hugging and it keeps the original shape of the candle intact.

Extinguishing style is important. A snuffer is recommended over blowing out the candle, apart from the annual birthday ritual, since snuffing does not release smoke into the air, which could challenge breathing.

Great caution should be taken with candle burning, however fragrant or festive, because it is a source of fire. The National Fire Incident Reporting System (NFIRS) reports that most fires caused by candles occur in the bedroom, followed by family room and bathroom. Most candle fire accidents occur when there is a problem with the holder; for example, when a candle-holder breaks or falls while the candle is still burning.

They advise people to refrain from touching burning candles or removing hot wax to avoid burns. NFIRS warns against candle burning when you are tired and likely to fall asleep, and they also advise against burning candles close to any heat source.[2]

Simmering Potpourri

In the olden days, women carried chafing dishes filled with steam-ing herbs and spices from room to room to freshen the air. Today, we continue this tradition with simmering potpourri. This recipe features herbs that are fragrant and antibacterial, antifungal, and antiviral to fight the germs that multiply and spread each winter.

To create a chafing dish of air-freshening simmering potpourri, mix and crumble by hand:

½ teaspoon each of organic rosemary, organic French lavender, organic lem-on eucalyptus, blue mallee eucalyptus, organic lemongrass, and organic peppermint essential oils (substitute with nonorganic, if need be).
2 cups dried rosemary
2 cups dried lavender
¾ cup dried eucalyptus leaves
½ cup dried peppermint
½ cup dried cedar tips
1 cup dried lemongrass
½ cup torn bay leaves

In a separate bowl blend:

1 cup orris root powder
1½ cup cellulose fiber

Mix the rosemary, French lavender, lemon eucalyptus, blue mallee eucalyptus, organic lemongrass, and peppermint essential oils in a non-reactive very small bowl, very gently. Set aside. While you breathe your healing energy into them, crumble the seven dried and torn herbs into a large nonreactive bowl. Add the mixed essential oils. Mix lovingly with your hands. Sprinkle on the orris root powder and cellulose fiber mixture. Stir together the entire mix with a stainless steel spoon or your clean, dry hands.

Store this essential oil and herbal blend with the preservatives in a large glass or stainless steel spring-top container away from light for three to four weeks.

Late December

Herbal Symbols of Winter

During winter, pagan beliefs, earth-based spirituality, and organized religion merge—particularly at Christmas. Numerous people celebrate the birth of Jesus Christ while others reflect on the symbolism of winter itself, beginning with the solstice. Winter is the special season for using frankincense and myrrh. These two resins speak of the golden spirit of redemption, protection, cleansing, and sharing gifts.

Frankincense and Myrrh

Frankincense and myrrh have a prominent role in African healing. These ancient resins have had folkloric, spiritual, and magical uses in the African diaspora as well. Frankincense and myrrh are holy incense to Hoodoos and practitioners of Santeria as well as Muslims, Catholics, Christians, and Jews.

Frankincense (*Boswellia sacra Flueck*): The resin was employed by the three wise men to honor the divinity of Jesus Christ. *Frank* means free, *incense* means lightning. The Arabic word for frankincense, *luban*, means "milk of the Arabs." Frankincense is celebrated as a perfume, incense, holy ointment, and superior fumigant. Frankincense is used heavily in the United States as spiritual incense and in blessing and anointment oil.

Myrrh (*Commiphora myrrha*): There are 135 species of myrrh growing in Africa and the Middle East—the highest grades were harvested in ancient Punt, modern day Somalia, and it is still harvested in this region today. Myrrh foretold the passion of the Christ. Heliopolis myrrh was burned at noon as incense for the ancient Egyptian sun god. Today, myrrh is widely enjoyed by Africans on the continent and within the diaspora. It is used in perfumery, as a scent for soap and other body care products, in certain foods (approved by FDA), and as a scent preservative. African American practitioners of Hoodoo use myrrh in blessing and anointment oils, along with frankincense. Myrrh is burned to honor the creator being and Great Mother figure, moon goddess Isis.

Myrrh Mouthwash

Myrrh is a natural mouth treatment used to treat serious gum diseases such as gingivitis and pyorrhea. Myrrh is also a healing medicine for cold sores and oral ulcers.

3 tablespoons myrrh
1 cup water
1 teaspoon 100-proof alcohol (vodka or gin)

Grind the myrrh finely using a mortar and pestle or a coffee grinder. Add to a pot with water. Cover. Heat on medium for twenty-five to thirty minutes. Strain. Pour through a funnel into a bottle. Add alcohol. Swirl to mix. Rinse mouth three times per day.

Spiritual Wash

Add eight drops frankincense and five drops myrrh to full bath. Chant or meditate. If you prefer, say a psalm or prayer of your choice.

Evergreens: Symbol of Life, Death, and Renewal

In African American tradition, evergreens are a metaphor for the interaction between departed spirits and the living community.

Evergreen Decoration

Bring the spirit of continuity, growth, and change into the home by collecting and displaying organic evergreens. Junipers with the berries are lovely. Holly with red berries is symbolic of the Holly King in western European traditions. Holly King is another name for the beloved

Father Winter and Father Christmas honored in England around Yule. A bouquet, spray, wreath, or garland featuring evergreens energizes the environment as well.

Evergreen Aromatherapy

If you become sick with a cold, bronchitis, or flu, be sure to add some of these greens to a pot of water. Decoct. Remove from heat, and tent with a towel by putting a clean bath towel over your head. Inhale the cleansing vapors designed to open up the nasal passages, bronchial system, and lungs, while also freeing up mucus.

Lift Me Up Pine Floor Wash

When I am cooped up indoors in the middle of winter, my spirits grieve the lively, spirited colors of autumn. Pine floor wash has a remarkable influence on the emotions. The floor wash below is recommended as a winter tonic for grief, mild depression, and fatigue. It is an updated formula featuring essential oils, and is antibiotic, antiseptic, and antifungal.

Fill a bucket three-fourths full of rainwater or spring water. Drop in essential oils, using a combination or a single oil: ¾ teaspoon of white pine (*Pinus sylvestris*) or ocean pine (*Pinus pinaster*), ½ teaspoon juniper (*Juniperus virginiana*), and ¼ teaspoon lemon (*Citrus limonum*) essential oils. Add three tablespoons of liquid Castile soap. Swirl the bucket gently to mix ingredients, focusing deeply on your healing intentions. Breathe deeply and slowly as you reflect over the water. Next grab a natural sea sponge, ordinary floor sponge, cotton rag, or your favorite mop. Scrub floors as you would with any other cleaning water, mopping surfaces thoroughly (don't wet floors excessively—use discretion or damage could occur as with any other heavy application of liquid to floors). Now, open the door or a window to release negative spirits and invite positive nature spirits. This also accelerates drying time.

Note: Test special types of wood or unusual floor covers for suitability before beginning. I have used this successfully on hardwood floors, tiles, and linoleum.

Pine infusion also makes a fine hair rinse or a mouthwash for sore throat and laryngitis. Chewing white pine refreshes breath; the needles contain vitamin C.

Corn and Kwanzaa: A Celebration of First Fruits

Throughout this book I speak of harvest of one type or another because it sets the tone for our seasonal activities. I also share folklore and celebrations involving the harvest. Throughout Africa (ancient and contemporary), harvest festivals have been a central feature of society.

Kwanzaa is a modern-day celebration developed in America in 1966 by Dr. Maulana Karenga, inspired by ancient traditions traced back to Nubia and Egypt, as well as the Swaziland empire, classical Ashantiland, and Yorubaland. Now, thanks to Dr. Karenga, Kwanzaa offers a unified way of observing community harvest during a single week across the globe.

Kwanzaa is Swahili for "first fruits," and it is a celebration of physical and spiritual harvesting. African Americans and all people can give thanks during Kwanzaa for all of the blessings bestowed upon them. Although Kwanzaa takes place from December 26–January 1, right in the heart of "shopping season," it is a holiday that shuns materialism and commercialism. Kwanzaa celebrates family, community, and holistic health, taking cues from traditional African society. In African culture, the anchors of society are the elders and the ancestors—nature is at the core of everyday life. Here are the principles and practices of Kwanzaa, written in Swahili first since it is the most widely spoken Pan-African language and because it is Karenga's preference as a way of discussing the holiday.

> › Nguzo Saba (en-goo-zo sah-bah): Seven Principles of Kwanzaa

> › Umoja (oo-moe-jah)—unity (December 26)

> › Kujichagulia (koo-jee-cha-goo-lee-ah)—self-determination (December 27)

> › Ujamaa (oo-jah-maah)—cooperative economics, fair trade, and supporting your community (December 28)

> › Ujima (oo-jee-mah)—collective work and responsibility (December 29)

> Kuumba (ku-oom-bah)—creativity (December 30)

> Nia (nee-ah)—purpose (December 31)

> Imani (ee-mahn-ee)—faith (January 1)

At the start of each of the days someone says, "*Habari gani*" (hah-bar-ee gah-nee), meaning "What is the news?" Reply by saying one of the Nguzo Sabo (seven principles). This reminds everyone of the theme for each day.

Red, black, and green are the official colors of this holiday. Red symbolizes the struggle of our people. Black stands for the African people. Green is hope and the future. A candleholder called a *kinara* (kee-nar-rah) is placed on a natural reed or straw mat called *mkeka* (em-kay-kah). The candles are placed as follows: the black candle, representing Umoja, is at the center. Three red candles representing Kujichagulia, Ujamaa, and Kuumba are placed to the left of the center candle. Three green candles representing Ujima, Nia, and Imani are placed to the right of the center candle. The black candle is lit the first day of Kwanzaa (December 26). Then each day thereafter, a new candle is lit, setting the tone to honor the theme of the day.

Dried corn is a "must-have" item for Kwanzaa. It is called *muhindi* (moo-hin-dee), meaning "crops," and at least two ears are placed on the mkeka. A large chalice called *kikombe cha umojo* (kee-kom-bay cha oo-moe-jah), or "Unity Cup" is placed on the mkeka as well. This is used to pour *tambiko* (libations) to the ancestors in remembrance and praise.

When celebrating Kwanzaa, be sure to invite friends and family to a potluck dinner. The preferred day for this is December 31, and it is called *karamu* (kaa-rah-moo) for "feast." Karamu with family is a way of maintaining relationships and building community essential to the holiday. As you bless the table, reflect upon the gifts of your ancestors. Family gifts are not a big priority, but they are sometimes given on January first and they are called *zawadi* (zah-wah-dee). Zawadi should be handmade or stimulating to the intellect. Apart from African arts and crafts, books are great zawadi.

Remember to eat the foods that enabled the ancestors to survive, because they continue to bless us with health. The colorful soul foods of our ancestors, rich in antioxidants and available during the winter include pumpkin; winter squash; collard, mustard, and turnip greens; rutabagas; turnips; parsnips; beets; oranges; and bananas. Make sure to include symbols of the harvest that are important to our African heritage on your Kwanzaa altar, including pumpkins, gourds, and dried corn. Kwanzaa can be confusing when you are first learning its traditions. Keep Kuumba in your heart, remember as many of the traditions as you can and then make the holiday your own.

Corn plays an important role in Kwanzaa and rightly so, as it has provided sustenance and nurturing in Africa and the diaspora for hundreds of years. For Native American nations, corn is a well-known, celebrated food with sacred significance. For example, the Algonquin people of the East Coast of the United States conceive of at least a quarter of their year using corn to name the full moons:

> › April is *Suquanni Kesos*—when they set the corn (planting corn moon)

> › May is *Moonesquanimock Kesos*—when women weed corn

> › August is *Micheenee Kesos*—when Indian corn is edible

> › September is *Phoquitaqunk Kesos*—the middle time between harvest and eating of Indian corn.

Corn Silk Tea

You can just imagine the first people coming across corn silk and thinking, *this is so gorgeous, surely it must have a use.* Indeed, corn silk is a useful herb and should not be thrown away. Corn silk is something that has often been overlooked. It is a kind friend to both elders and children. Corn silk is a diuretic that helps condition the bladder and reduce bedwetting. It is particularly helpful to seniors because it helps diminish build-up of solids that restrict the flow of urine. Corn silk helps to heal numerous ailments and malfunctions of the bladder including inflammation that also affects the kidneys and urethra. Corn silk is used as a folk cure for high blood pressure, to lower cholesterol, and to treat arteriosclerosis.

Shuck two ears of corn; reserve shucks and corn for other projects. Bring water to simmer. Add corn silk. Cover, reduce heat to medium, and infuse for ten minutes. Strain and drink. You can follow this same procedure to make a hair conditioner. Instead of drinking it, let it cool and then use it as a final rinse to soften the hair.

Succotash #1

My mother and aunt would make this dish in a seasoned cast iron skillet and you might like to try it as well. Cast iron can supply small amounts of iron in the diet, especially when using a recipe like this one that contains tomato or other acidic fruit.

Shuck six ears of corn. Remove silk, and set it aside for other projects. Hold corn at a slight angle pressed to the cutting board. With a very sharp carving knife, cut the corn going with the grain over the cutting board. Mince a small onion. Remove the seeds and interior from a green, yellow, red, or orange pepper. Cut in half. Mince the pepper. Cube two tomatoes. Sauté in one teaspoon olive or corn oil (using a spraying oil is fine). Add sea salt and freshly ground pepper. Add a dash of cayenne or hot sauce if a spicy taste is desired.

Succotash #2

My Aunt Edith, a family elder who was married to a Native American named Uncle Henry, taught me to make this. It is a simple recipe that we enjoyed as children, during the cool days of fall and winter:

I-Ya-Tsu-Ya-Di-Su-Yise-Lu (also called Cherokee Succotash) is hearty enough to serve as a soup meal with corn bread on the side or as tasty side dish. This recipe can be performed over an open fire as readily as it can be done indoors on the stove.

    2 cups lima beans (dried)
    8 cups water
    4 cups corn fresh from cob
    1 onion (wild if possible)
    1 tablespoon butter
    1½ teaspoons sea salt, divided

1 teaspoon peppercorns
1 teaspoon sugar
4 cups free-range chicken stock
1 pound bear meat, a ham hock, or 2 turkey drumsticks
1 cup cream (optional)

Wash limas; pick out undesirable beans or debris if any. Put the limas in a pot of water (a cast iron Dutch oven or other heavy-bottomed pot works well). Add ½ teaspoon sea salt. Bring to a boil. Cover. Remove from heat, and let stand one hour (set timer). Meanwhile, shuck the corn. Store the corn silk for later use as medicinal tea (see page 57) or hair rinse. Cut corn kernels from the ears with a sharp knife following the directions from Succotash #1. Put the corn kernels and corn milk aside in a large bowl. Finely mince the onion. Place the butter in a cast iron skillet over medium-high heat. Sprinkle with the remaining sea salt. Add freshly ground black pepper (not traditional, but tasty all the same). Sprinkle one teaspoon of sugar over the onion and spices. Add corn. Cook 'til lightly browned. Once the timer goes off, rinse limas and put them back into the pot. Cover with the chicken stock. Add the ingredients of the skillet to the pot along with the meat of your choice. Simmer two hours on medium heat or until meat is tender. Stir in cream. Simmer on low, fifteen minutes or so to warm thoroughly.

Serve hot.

Thanks, Aunt Edith and Uncle Henry, R.I.P!

January 1, New Year's—Winter Spirit: Inspiration and Renewal

New Year's Eve is a time to look back on the previous year. We reflect on good times and bad, we mourn those whom we have lost as we make way for the new life ahead. New Year's Day is the time many of us choose to make resolutions for how to be better people in the coming year. The New Year is a time when we can seek luck to have a prosperous, healthy, and abundant year. Traditionally we include symbolic foods including black-eyed peas, white rice, stewed tomato, and collard greens.

Hoppin' John

1 pound black-eyed peas, dry
1½ tablespoons olive oil (or spray)
1 large onion
1 green pepper
2 cloves garlic
Pinch sea salt
½ teaspoon freshly ground peppercorns
½ teaspoon cumin, ground
Pinch dried cayenne pepper spice
24 ounces organic free-range chicken broth or vegetable broth
2 cups chopped tomato

Pick over and remove debris or damaged peas. Soak the black-eyed peas overnight in a bowl, or follow the quick-cooking directions on the package. Discard the water and rinse (this reduces the tendency for the beans to give gastric distress). Add oil to a Dutch oven or stockpot. Set heat at medium. Mince onion, green pepper, and garlic cloves finely, keeping each separate. Sauté the onion until translucent. Add green pepper, sauté five minutes, then stir in garlic and continue cooking. Add spices; stir to mix all ingredients well. Pour in broth; stir well. Cover. Simmer on low for a half hour. Add chopped tomato; cover again. Cook until beans are soft and tender. Test; add more spices if desired.

Stewed Tomato

3 cups chopped tomato
1 tablespoon white sugar
Pinch fine sea salt
¼ teaspoon white peppercorns, finely ground
Slice of French bread
1 tablespoon unsalted butter

Add tomato to a cast iron or other pot. Turn heat to low. Add the next three ingredients and stir. Cube bread and add it and the butter. Cook gently for thirty minutes.

Collard Greens

1 pound of collard greens
5 strips bacon
1 Spanish onion
3 cloves garlic
1 teaspoon cayenne pepper
1 teaspoon sea salt
1½ teaspoons black peppercorns, ground
¼ cup apple cider vinegar
32 ounces organic free-range turkey broth
2 free range smoked turkey drumsticks or wings

Sort the collard greens. Discard yellow, brown, or badly damaged leaves. Soak the greens in a sink or deep basin of cold water for thirty minutes to remove soil. Cut the bacon into half-inch squares, and fry it in a Dutch oven or other heavy-bottomed pot on medium-high heat for three minutes. Chop the onion finely and add it to the bacon, stir, and sauté until the onion is transparent. Mince garlic, and add it along with the cayenne pepper, salt, and ground pepper. Cook three more minutes. Add vinegar to deglaze the pan. Stir; simmer about five minutes. Strain greens; chop coarsely. Add the greens, broth, and turkey. Reduce the heat to medium. Cook for about two and a half to three hours, until the greens and turkey are soft and tender. Check the seasonings—add more if desired. Remove meat from cartilage and bones. Discard the bones. Serve the greens with a little turkey and a small amount of broth. This can be a meal in itself or it can be served along with other soul foods during the holidays. The broth is called "pot liquor" and can be consumed, sipped in a cup separately. This is especially good when fighting a cold or building immunity.

White Rice

2 cups white rice
4 cups water or broth
1 tablespoon oil (corn, canola, olive)
Pinch of fine sea salt

Add ingredients to a rice cooker and cook. If no rice cooker is available, add all ingredients to an appropriately sized pot. Stir. Set heat at medium-high. Once ingredients come to a boil, cover and set heat at the lowest possible setting. Cook twenty to twenty-five minutes until all the liquid is absorbed. Do not stir; don't peek if you can help it. Taking these steps greatly helps ensure the success of a well-cooked pot of rice.

Though brown rice can certainly be substituted as it is healthier and preferred by some, white rice has been traditionally used by African Americans and Afro-Cubans. It is the rice our people helped cultivate during enslavement and beyond in North Carolina and its environs. The white rice also has a symbolic meaning, standing for male fertility, whereas the red tomato symbolizes female fertility. The combination of Hoppin' John, stewed tomato, collard greens, and white rice is believed to bring in good luck. This was typically served with some type of pork. Recipes for a variety of ways to cook pork can be found online.

Carnations and the Feast of Aphrodite

Sometime during the first week of January, the feast of Greek love goddess, Aphrodite, is celebrated. Prepare for a feast honoring Aphrodite's loving sensuality and warmth. Decorate with pink carnations; they are the flowers of friendship. Burn warm yellow sandalwood-scented candles—sandalwood loosens inhibitions. Put symbols of love including pomegranates, apples, and seashells out in blue ceramic or crystal bowls. Invite friends to bring an aphrodisiac food for sharing (cherries, oysters, papaya, chocolate, truffles, red wine, etc.). Open a window or door slightly. Join hands around the dinner table.

Recite this invocation:

> *Aphrodite, Greek goddess of friendship, love, and life*
> *Come join us, bring peace, and eliminate all strife*
> *We welcome you with fruit, flowers, fire, and fresh air*
> *Release us from anxiety, stress, or despair*

Come down; be with us
Grace us this special day
We call you with love
We hope you will stay

Repeat three times, with sincerity.

February 14, Saint Valentine's Day—
Making Way for Winter Romance

Saint Valentine's Day is a time to revel in the decadence of romance and love in its many different manifestations. Sweet smelling flowers and comfort foods are featured treats, as are aphrodisiacs like chocolate, fresh fruit, and gifts of the sea. Shrouding ourselves in warmth and comfort provides a respite from winter, affording an opportunity to nourish the mind, body, and spirit. In the home spa, we tenderly care for dry skin, hair, and nails with herbs and natural oils at a fraction of the cost of commercial spas.

The Rose (*Rosa* spp.)

No other plant is as intimately linked with love as the rose. When selecting healing roses, seek out the old-fashioned scented types such as those listed below, rather than the more neutral tea roses:

Apothecary's Rose: the fragrant rose from which a very high quality of rose water is made.

Belle de Crecy: considered by some to contain the purest rose scent.

Celestial: a rose with a crisp and clean aroma.

Kazanlik: a Bulgarian rose oil also called attar of roses is made from this rose. It throws off a potent smell I consider very heady.

Madame Isaac Pereire, **Guinee**, and **Souvenir de la Malmaison:** are stunning and highly fragrant.

Maiden's Blush: is considered to be a more refined scent.

Roses are beautiful, and like the lotus, they suggest female genitalia in the height of passion. The blush of the rose is often compared to the blush of a bride or a sexual partner during orgasm. In parts of Africa and the Middle East, holy temples are spiritually cleansed entirely with highly potent Bulgarian rose water typically called rose hydrosol or simple rose water. Rose hydrosol enhances the sacred environment.

A little-known fact is that roses are a systemic nervine—translation: they calm and soothe your nerves. Fresh roses, rose water, rose otto (attar of roses), rose cream, and rose incense all cast a magical spell, binding love and romance. The following recipes feature high fragrance and the ubiquitous food of the gods—ingredients with a time-honored tradition in love magic cross-culturally.

Neroli Affirmations

After the flurry of holidays, sometimes there is a downturn in mood by the time Valentine's Day rolls around. This is multiplied if you are single, on the verge of a breakup, or widowed. These affirmations are useful healers for a variety of reasons. Are you sick of seeing and smelling roses this time of the year? Try neroli absolute or essential oil—it is a spiritual oil that builds confidence where it is lacking and cheers up the spirit. You can do this in three different ways, depending on what is available to you:

1. Place a bowl of fresh oranges you have carefully selected on a piece of furniture or on the sink near a mirror.

2. Dab neroli oil (sparingly) on your pulse points (temple, wrists, back of the knees, etc.).

3. Mist your face and hair with neroli hydrosol (also called orange flower water) then say each affirmation as you look in the mirror.

   I accept myself as I am

   I welcome the person I am becoming

   I surround myself with love

I forgive myself for the mistakes I have made
I forgive the harm brought to me by others
I am ready to move forward

Blessed Be!

Romantic Flower Projects for St. Valentine's Day

› Pink carnations suggest enduring friendship, warmth, and trust. They are inexpensive, even in the winter, and add a nice touch to a romantic dinner.

› Buy fragrant old-fashioned flowers of your favorite scent and color.

› Peel petals away from organic fragrant flowers (roses work well). Float these in a bath for two. Light vanilla-scented candles for a pleasant accent.

› Sprinkle rose petals on your mattress, under your bed, on your bed, in your closets, in your purse and any place where the compassionate spirit of the rose is desired.

› For a sexy bath, add ¼ cup of rose water to one cup of milk. Stir in eight drops jasmine absolute and 4 drops each of lotus and patchouli oils. Mist your wet body (bodies) after a bath or shower with fragrant neroli hydrosol, also called orange flower water.

› Put a fragrant gardenia or lily in your hair before going out to a party or on a date.

› Mist face and hair with lavender hydrosol before leaving home—especially if inhibitions and tension are coming between you and finding love.

› Set out seven to nine lit candles scented with a relaxing essential oil such as neroli, sandalwood, chamomile, or lavender, in the room where you will entertain your company.

› Old-fashioned stock flower and delphinium in blues, whites, and lavender are warming and invite a long, steady relationship.

Saint Valentine's Day Love Potion and Meditation

Collect yourself. Breathe deeply and evenly. Focus on your intentions for love and a healthy relationship as you collect the following ingredients:

2 cups high quality dry red wine
2 slices orange
1 (8-inch) cinnamon stick
⅛ teaspoon allspice
2 cracked white cardamom pods
⅛ teaspoon ground ginger
Drop of your blood (optional)

Take a cleansing breath (inhalation) and visualize your passion pouring out into a pot as you exhale. Your intention becomes the first ingredient. Pour wine into the pot. Cut the orange slices in half and add. Break the cinnamon stick. Stir in spices and blood (if adding, use a sterilized needle). Heat on medium-low until warm but not boiling. Let the mixture cool slightly. Pour into glasses. Drink with your intended.

Chocolate Soap

Some soap makers, this one included, tend to get carried away with the chocolate soap theme, especially during the winter holidays. Using soap molds creatively adds even more fun. Molds used for chocolate making can easily be used to create soap. (Just pour the freshly made soap into chocolate molds, as you would use any other mold.) Sun-Feather Natural Soap Company produces heavenly scented chocolate fragrance oil that can be used alone or in combination with a variety of oils to carry through the chocolate theme. Orange, lemon, or cassia essential oils work well also with handmade cocoa butter products. Vanilla or coconut fragrance oils compliment chocolate soap. Chocolate-colored soap poured into chocolate molds can then be put into heart-shaped or other traditional chocolate boxes as a novel St. Valentine's treat.

Chocolate Soap

4.5 ounces goat milk
10 ounces distilled water
5 ounces lye
12 ounces vegetable shortening
8 ounces tallow
12 ounces coconut oil
2 ounces unsweetened Baker's chocolate
Vegetable cooking spray
1 ounce cocoa butter

Freeze milk the night before soapmaking. Thaw milk in the morning. Measure all ingredients on a scale. Put on goggles, an apron, and plastic gloves for protection. Mix milk and water in a quart-sized Pyrex liquid measuring cup. Stir in lye using a stainless steel spoon. Set aside.

Melt all fats (except cocoa butter) and chocolate in stainless steel stockpot on medium heat. Remove from heat. Using a meat thermometer, take the temperature of oils and water/milk mix (clean thermometer after it is used for the oils so it doesn't contaminate the water/milk mixture). Spray the soap mold(s). Set aside. Melt cocoa butter in the microwave, stovetop, or regular oven. Set aside. When both sets of ingredients equal 120 degrees, slowly stir milk/water mixture into oils with the stainless steel spoon. Continue to stir with a "figure eight" motion. Chocolate soap is ready to pour into soap or candy molds or a rectangular Pyrex casserole dish when you drizzle a portion on top of the batch and it retains its shape—this is called trace. When soap reaches trace, stir in the melted cocoa butter, then pour it into the molds. Cover immediately with wool blankets. Do not disturb. After twenty-four hours, remove the blankets. Soap solidifies after forty-eight to sixty-four hours; when solid, remove it from the mold(s). If using a casserole dish, measure out 2 x 3-inch bars that will resemble brownies. Set on shelves, away from direct heat or sunlight, for four to six weeks. Scrape residue off the bottom of a bar with a sharp knife; use the knife to bevel edges for a very neat look. Wrap the soap in cellophane or put it inside decorative boxes.

CHAPTER FIVE

Spiritual Warmth, Good Health, and Immunity

Teatime

Winter is a time when we seek warmth in all of its variations—spiritual warmth, protection from the cold, nourishment of friendship and family. Many people suffer from depression during the winter because of the fact that there is less daylight. Specific herbs possess warming ways, which insulate the body and spirit from the harsh aspects of winter. For those desiring warming herbal infusions, here are some ideas to get you started.

Making Tea

Tea is an herbal infusion also called a tisane. Sometimes tough herbs are decocted and taken as tea as well. Honey, lemon, and tea go together well. Milk (not cream) and honey are also pleasant accompaniments to full-bodied teas. I always recommend using certified organic honey, especially if you are using it medicinally.

To make a good cup of tea, you need patience. Add cold water to the kettle. Boil water; turn off heat. Pour some into clean tea cup(s) and let it sit three to five minutes. Pour this water out into a plugged kitchen sink for washing up later. Add tea bags or infusers with herbs inside (usually about a single teaspoon to a cup of water) to cups. Pour very hot water from the teakettle into a cup until it is three quarters full. Steep at least five minutes, longer for a stronger brew. Remove the tea bag or infuser. Drink as is or add what you prefer.

Black Tea, Green Tea, and Oolong *(Camellia sinensis)*
Tea is one of the oldest natural remedies known to man. Legend has it that a fresh leaf from *Camellia sinensis* fell from a tree and into the Chinese emperor's pot that was boiling water outside. He was intrigued by the smell, tasted it, and enjoyed it immensely; then he made it a regular habit to consume this as tea. The type of tea the emperor made by mistake is commonly called green tea since it was made from fresh green leaves. Green tea is a very strong medicinal tea, as is oolong, and black tea. Green tea contains antioxidants that are believed to be two hundred times stronger than vitamin E. Green tea protects the cells from carcinogens—the substance responsible is catekin. Catekin lowers cholesterol, metabolizes fat, reduces blood pressure, regulates blood sugar, and has an antibacterial action. Green tea, and all tea for that matter, helps teeth and gums stay healthy. Green tea contains fluoride. It also helps with bronchial infections and mild respiratory ailments, as well as asthma and breathing difficulties. Black teas are fermented, creating numerous strong dark-colored teas. In China, these teas are called oolongs, while in India the favorite tea is black assam. There are more than three thousand varieties of tea created from *Camellia sinensis*.

Rooibos: the Cure-all of South Africa
Annemarie Fillmore-Nava hails from Cape Town, South Africa, and is a descendant of the Zulu people. In this interview, she fondly recalls what the tea meant to her growing up and why she now gives it to her young son as a preferred beverage:

First a pronunciation key—in South Africa we spell the name of this herb "rooibos" or "rooibosch," but it is more commonly called "bossie." Bossie is pronounced as if "o" is a "oa" sound, as in coat. Bossie tea has been a staple in my life ever since I was a young child. Not only is it a common drink in South Africa because it is native to our land, but also because of the health properties. The Adventist Church, of which I was a member growing up, follows a very regimented diet abstaining from pork, shellfish, alcohol, and caffeine, among others. Bossie is the preferred hot beverage for most Seventh-day Adventists because it fits into our beliefs about health and spirituality. It contains no tannin or caffeine and is renowned for immune-boosting properties. It is a very versatile herbal tea in that you can drink it with or without milk. You can buy it loose-leaf or already in teabags; either way is fine, although we found the bags to be more convenient. It has a very clean, naturally sweet taste to it and such a beautiful red colour.

Whenever we had a cold, my mother would say, "I know what you need, you need some bossie tea with lemon and honey. That will get you better in no time." And that is exactly what she would give us. Because this tea is so pure, you can give it to babies who have colic. In that case you simply give it to them plain. Plain meaning no milk or sugar (older children through adults usually drink it with milk and sugar—also called "English style"). Bossie really doesn't require sugar because it has a naturally sweet taste. Infants will gladly accept this tea because of its naturally mild sweetness.

We also use it for children or adults who have diarrhea as it settles the stomach. Again, it would be served plain. This tea is also used as an appetite stimulant, so during recovery from an illness when you need to eat but just can't seem to, a cup of plain bossie tea will do the job. Needless to say, it is not a dieter's tea. However, this drink is great for those nights that you just can't seem to relax. The best way to serve it for this purpose is to brew the bags with milk on the stove. When you use only milk with it, it has a very creamy texture and really warms your insides, much like the effects of hot chocolate on a cold day.

Many a day in the winter we would play in the rain and come inside to a warm milk and bossie drink. There were five of us coming at different times to make our tea so my mother would often be very irritated with us as children, because as you well know what happens to milk when it comes to a boil—it boils over. I can still hear her saying, "I just cleaned the stove. Who made bossie tea and did not clean the stove?" I always remember standing in front of the stove waiting for that boiling point so that I would not have to clean the stove. My brother never learnt that trick so he was always stuck cleaning the stove.

Besides the medicinal purposes, this is just a great all-around drinking tea. One does not need any specific reason other than you would like a hot beverage to drink. In South Africa, we drink our tea typically with milk and sugar. Even though we drink a lot of English tea for enjoyment, I continue to use this tea for my son who is six years old. He has been drinking this tea since he was born for all of the reasons and purposes I spoke about. He absolutely loves it and drinks it with milk or plain, but usually with milk. As we all sit around drinking tea, he desperately wanted to be included in this ritual, so this was and is a wonderful replacement for teatime with kids because of the absence of caffeine and the absolute clean sweet taste. If you are looking for a tea to enjoy that also has excellent health properties, this is the one.

We also use this tea as a first aid for wounds and cuts. In this case we use loose-leaf and make a paste with water, which is applied directly to the wound. It draws out any infection. So as you can see, it is our cure-all. Thanks to the Khoisan people who discovered it and its many uses ages ago.

Rooibos (*Aspalathus linearis*): grows exclusively in the Clanwilliam district of the Western Cape of South Africa,[2] where the age-old tradition of wildcrafting the organic herb continues. It is truly a remarkable red medicine. Rooibos contains fifty times more antioxidants than green tea. It contains a free radical damage scavenger, super oxide dismatase (SOD). SOD helps keep fat from turning into harmful lipid peroxide. Quercetin, a flavanol, brings the greatest gift to our blood, lending the tea the ability to prevent hemorrhaging, increase circulation, build capillary strength, as well as fight infections.[3] Rooibos mineral counts, per 200 milliliters tea:

Calcium 1.09 mg
Copper 0.07 mg
Fluoride 0.22 mg
Iron 0.07 mg
Manganese 0.04 mg
Magnesium 1.57 mg
Sodium 6.16 mg
Zinc 0.04[4]

When seeking antioxidants and health tonic, reach for rooibos or green tea.

Roman Chamomile (*Anthemis nobilis*) (*Chamaemelum nobile*)
German Chamomile (*Matricaria chamomile*) (*Matricaria recutita*)
One of the most relaxing teas is made from perky yellow chamomile flower. Chamomile tea reduces aches, strains, arthritis, and menstrual cramps. It helps reduce bladder infections and reduces the presence of *E. coli* in the bladder. Chamomile also soothes the stomach and reduces vomiting. It is an all purpose soother that calms, cools, and tranquilizes, helping you relax and sleep better. It calms the digestive tract and reduces abdominal pain, bloating, and gas.

With these excellent choices to choose from, what could be better than a tea party?

Osayin Tea Party
Winter is an excellent time of the year to invoke the orisha Osayin. Osayin tried to hide all the herbal knowledge he possessed inside a gourd hung high in a tree so the other orishas wouldn't be able to use it. The gourd fell down to earth, teaching us that herbal knowledge is not to be rarified or secreted away, but shared by all. Despite his naughty history, Osayin is the patron orisha of herbalism.

With all the talk about tea, one of the world's most commonly used herbs, today is as good a day as any to have an herbal tea party. Select some of the herbal kingdom's most powerful healing teas to share.

Choose from one of the superb herbals just discussed: black tea (loose leaf Darjeeling, Earl Grey, Ceylon, oolong, or a choice Russian would be suitable for a tea party), your favorite green tea (again loose and unflavored to savor the true essence of this healing tea), rooibos, or the peace-inducing chamomile flower tea.

One teaspoon per cup of hot water will suffice. Add the loose tea to a tea ball, muslin tea bag, or bamboo tea strainer for convenience. This way there won't be any stray leaves in your brew. Sweeten with honey if desired. Try a flavored honey, such as lavender or rose honey, to add a special touch.

Go English-style by adding a bit of milk; this makes tea almost like a dessert. This is appropriate with the Indian teas (Darjeeling, Ceylon, or Earl Grey) enjoyed in England. Try it Eastern European-styled with a slice of lemon for a refreshing taste that renews energy. Tea with lemon is preferred for full-bodied black teas such as the Russian type. Green tea, oolong, and chamomile are wonderful on their own without any special enhancements. Rooibos is naturally sweet and rich enough to be lightened with a bit of milk.

Use a special cup—handmade earthenware, which speaks so well of the union of hand, fire, and earth, is the ideal choice. You will find these at art or craft fairs and specialty shops, unless you happen to make them yourself. After your tea is made, shake a gourd rattle over your guests' heads as you sing praise to each person:

> *I give this to you in good health Blessings*
>
> *Herbal knowledge is free Blessings*
>
> *Praise Osayin Blessings*
>
> *Praise Mother Earth Blessings!*

Sweeten tea with honey if desired. Enjoy the fellowship of your circle on this feast day of Osayin.

Oats (*Avena sativa*)

I consider oats soul food, since they nourish and comfort on a level that goes beyond physical hunger. Oat straw provides a protective energy by strengthening our inner core. Oatmeal and oat straw are natural remedies for stress that manifests as headaches, insomnia, and itchy skin. Full baths of oatmeal or oat straw soak away emotional stress and physical pain by penetrating the outer layers of skin. Soaking a cloth in oat water and applying it to the face reduces the appearance of wrinkles and keeps the skin supple and glowing. Following are three recipes featuring ways to use oats during the winter season:

Oat Bath #1

> Large stockpot
> Enough steel-cut oats to cover bottom
> Water

Cover the bottom of the stockpot with oats. Fill the pot three-fourths full of water. Boil. Turn down to medium-low and cook for several hours. The film that develops on top is an emollient, useful for treating dry itchy skin. Apply this directly to dry areas using a cotton square or facecloth. After a few hours, strain the oats through a wire-mesh colander lined with cheesecloth. Take a bowl of the hot oat milk to bathroom; add to a tub of warm water. Soak for at least twenty minutes.

Oat Bath #2

> 1 half-gallon jar
> 2 ounces dried oat straw
> Water

Bring water and oat straw close to boiling. Cover. Reduce heat to low. Steep four hours. Strain. Add two cups to hot bath.

Oat Bath #3

Place several ounces of oats in a washcloth. Gather all four corners together and secure with a rubber band. Suspend it with string from the faucet of hot running water in your bath. As you bathe, squeeze washcloth of oat bath to your face. Apply this to your hair and scalp as well—it is especially useful for winter dryness and eczema.

Fragrant Woods

Quite naturally, we gravitate toward the light as the days grow shorter. Here are a few suggestions for using the element of fire (smoldering wood) to scent the winter home. Aromatic woods for the fire include cedar, eucalyptus, juniper, pine, cedar, apple, and balsam poplar. Most any herb can be added to a fire, particularly as the fire is almost dying out. Fragrant herbs for the fire include mugwort, lavender, juniper, sage, spearmint, rosemary, and lemon verbena.

Incense

Incense is a wonderful alternative to larger fires for those living in a home without a fireplace; it can even be used in small, confined spaces such as efficiency apartments and dorm rooms—though good ventilation is required. There are incense recipes dispersed throughout the book; frankincense, myrrh, and a recipe for release incense are included in this chapter. The following five ingredients are especially magical used alone or added to more elaborate incense blends.

Aloeswood (*Aquilaria agallocha*): is the jewel of the East, but it is something we here in the West might not be too familiar with. Take it from me, treat yourself—this is sultry, exotic, and unique. It is also a very relaxing wood. Aloeswood, or *oud* as it is sometimes called, is one of the most sought-after aromatic woods on Earth.

Cedarwood chips (*Cedrus libani or C.* spp.): On the other side of the coin is the very common cedarwood. Cedarwood is sold at pet stores as bedding for small animals and is widely available (if you have a wood shop you might even have your own). As an easily grown tree in the United States, cedar has been a highly touted aromatic wood used in sacred ceremonies by various Native American tribes for centuries. Cedar incense is complex, and it is a great spiritual cleansing smoke. The incense is said to cure head colds and the tendency to have bad dreams.

Cinnamon (*Cinnamomum verum, C. zeylanicum*): Usually sold in sticks made from quills of the inner bark. Cinnamon burns easily and releases a spicy scent into the air. It is considered a protective smoke capable of encouraging high spiritual vibrations and aiding healing.

Nag Champa (*Michelia champaca*): Comes from India, and it is one of the most popular types of incenses. Traditionally used by the Hindi and Buddhists for meditation and temple rites, nag champa is a relaxing, inexpensive, widely available, ready-made, multipurpose, spiritual incense. (Usually sold as prepared incense, not loose.)

Sandalwood (*Santalum album*): Though sandalwood hails from India, the three-hundred-year-old Baieido Company from Japan makes choice incense from sandalwood chips. Sandalwood is considered an aphrodisiac that builds self-confidence and generates well-being within the environment. Sandalwood blends well with any of the incense herbs listed in this section and with frankincense and myrrh.

Fragrant woods are sold already prepared as stick or cone incense and sometimes loose, sold by weight. To begin, experiment with fragrant woods and spices, broken into small pieces. Choose from this list of woods: aloeswood (oud), cedarwood, cinnamon bark, eucalyptus, juniper, pine, cedar, apple, and balsam poplar. The herbs include mugwort, lavender, juniper, white sage, mint, rosemary, and lemon verbena. Make your selections, mix, and then burn on a white-hot bamboo charcoal that is placed on a fireproof burner. You can also add pinches of these to a wood-burning fire. Make sure you have good ventilation for whichever way you decide to use incense.

Spiritual Essential Oils, Floral Waters, and Absolutes

Full submission to the home, community, and family is greatly enhanced by re-engagement with herbs and deity. The following herbs have strong spiritual energy, and many of them assist with prayer and invocation of specific goddesses. Here are a few useful herbs, flowers, and resins, with qualities that enhance spiritual communion during the winter.

Carnation Absolute (*Dianthus caryophyllus*): purportedly the actual fragrance of angels, fresh carnations or carnation absolute encourages friendship, nurtures relationships, and creates an inviting atmosphere. Carnations are useful during tarot card readings and other forms of divination as the scent encourages prophetic dreams and brings us to a higher plane than where we normally exist. Only one drop of carnation absolute should be added to the bath, dream pillow, sachet, potpourri, or other botanical, as it is very potent.

Champa (*Michelia champaca*): (syn. Nag Champa) Nag champa has a delightful scent that is relaxing yet energizing to the spirit. Champa is a perfectly balanced aroma, believed to inspire happiness. Nag champa is widely available as incense from Thailand.

Frankincense (*Boswellia sacra, Boswellia* spp.): is a symbol of divinity. Considered sacred incense, it is often utilized for meditation, prayer, invocation, and healing. Frankincense is considered a protective resin and it dispels fear. Try a frankincense smoke bath outdoors. Burn a few resins at a time on a charcoal block on a fireproof surface; pull the smoke overhead with your hands.

Jasmine (*Jasminum officinale*): is a high frequency, sweet, romantic scent that eases anxiety and aids sleep. Jasmine is one of the *ewe* (herbs) of Yemaya, thus it is thought of as a maternal, kind, caring, and instructive herb that is great for dreaming and vision quests. Try adding a teaspoon of dried flowers to a cup of very hot water sweetened with honey as a bedtime tea. Jasmine is a wonderful addition to dream pillows, and it can be used as a scent for powder, candles, sachets, or food for a mojo bag.

Lavender (*Lavandula angustifolia*): is a hard worker. It calms, balances, and was considered an aphrodisiac by early Western herbalists; it is used by Hoodoos to attract those of the same sex. Lavender soothes and comforts. Fill a spray bottle with lavender water, use it to charge your altar space, home, or work environment and spray it on your hair, face, and body to revive your spirit. The essential oil can be used externally, neat. Lavender is a wonderful scent for handmade furniture polish and as a spiritual floor wash.

Lemongrass (*Cymbopogon citrates, C. flexuosus*): is an energizing spirit lifter. Burn lemongrass with lavender, sandalwood, and cedar chips or with crushed frankincense and myrrh. Add ½ teaspoon lemongrass to a bucket of soapy water; use it as a spiritual floor wash or house cleanser.

Lotus (*Nelumbo nucifera*): Lotus is considered a representative of the divine feminine and the embodiment of Tehuti in Egyptian tradition. The scent is moist and watery, suggestive of the fecundity of the Great Earth Mother. Lotus oil comes from blue, white, and pink flowers—each has a distinctive scent: blue or white is great for an introduction to lotus. Pink lotus flowers represent Lakshmi Devi, goddess of prosperity to the Hindi. Dab lotus oil onto pulse points, the chakras, or add a few drops to the bath. It is a very sensual, unusual oil.

Myrrh (*Commiphora erythraea*): Break off about ½ teaspoon myrrh from larger block—it breaks easily with a mallet. Burn the myrrh on a charcoal block in the same manner as frankincense—myrrh and frankincense are usually combined for a more spiritually balancing blend with ⅔ frankincense to ⅓ myrrh because of myrrh's high strength.

Combined myrrh and frankincense represent Yoruban orisha Egungun-Oya, arbitrator of destiny and fate, as well as facilitator of communication with ancestors. Add 3 to 4 drops myrrh to bath, or use it neatly, dabbed on the pulse points or chakras.

Note: if you are pregnant, check with your health practitioner before using myrrh.

Rose Otto (*Rosa damascena*): Whatever you need—calm, balance, stimulation, an aphrodisiac, cooling off after an argument—rose otto or attar of roses can help. Bulgarian roses are widely available in East Indian shops and health food stores, prepared as a rose water that can be put into a spray bottle. Rose water is considered cleansing, a blessing oil that also purifies the environment. Rose otto is very expensive but it is also very powerful—a few drops will do the trick! Add two drops to a full bath, to a dream pillow, sachet, or mojo bag. Roses are associated with a variety of love goddesses including the orisha Oshun and Greek goddess Aphrodite. White roses are associated with the tears of the Roman goddess Venus. Pink roses suggest the perfume of Erzulie Freda in Haitian Vodou.

Note: Pregnant women should avoid the use of rose otto.

Sandalwood (*Santalum album*): the mellow scent of sandalwood eases inhibitions, builds self-confidence, induces a calm, sedate mood, and can assist in achieving a meditative state. Sandalwood is considered an aphrodisiac—fittingly, it is also an ewe (herb) of orisha Oshun. It is wonderful when applied to the body as a massage oil, diluted with sweet almond oil; ½ teaspoon sandalwood essential oil to eight ounces of sweet almond. It can also be applied to pulse points or chakras neatly before going out or at bedtime. Baieido sandalwood incense is a high grade and fine cut suitable for mixing with other incense ingredients or burning on a charcoal block alone.

CHAPTER SIX

Immunity and Nervous System

Tea for Colds, Flu, Depression, Aches, and Pains

One of the major drawbacks to winter is the profusion of germs passing from one person to the next, sparking colds and influenza. To make matters worse, African Americans are disproportionately afflicted by upper respiratory illnesses like asthma and bronchitis, as well as compromised immune systems. The following herbs allow you to tap into the healing energy of the earth's plants and trees to fight ailments that strike frequently during winter. These herbs and natural ingredients have a history of helping us build immunity.

Camphor Tree *(Cinnamomum camphora)*

Camphor leaves have a clean-smelling scent reminiscent of mothballs. Camphor is used medicinally, particularly in Chinese medicine where it is called *Hsiang Chang*. The Chinese prize this substance as a treatment for heart ailments, circulatory problems, and as a digestive. Camphor is used as a sedative and calming agent and to treat convulsions, hysteria, and insomnia. In the West, we have concentrated on using camphor to treat the discomforts of cold and flu, upper respiratory ailments, rheumatism, muscle pains, and body aches. Camphorated oil, Grandma's favorite, can be made by adding a few drops of the essential oil to three tablespoons melted aloe butter, shea butter, or mango butter. You can also add a drop or so of camphor oil to a handkerchief and inhale the scent to clear nasal passages and sinuses. (You can use eucalyptus similarly to camphor; see below.)

Wild camphor tree *(Tarchonanthus camphorates)*
Several South African companies sell bush teas internationally (wild-crafted, organic, indigenous herbs) that contain wild camphor. Wild camphor tree offers many benefits. The South African Khoisan people use wild camphor for its soothing qualities. Dried leaves are used in ceremonies to anoint the body during rituals. The leaves and seeds are used to fumigate. Camphor smoke treats rheumatism, headache, and insomnia. The tea relieves stomach ailments, asthma, anxiety, and heartburn. The leaves contain an insecticide used to deter lice and external parasites.

Echinacea *(Echinacea angustifolia)*

Echinacea roots, flowers, and stems have been used traditionally as an antiseptic, as a blood purifier, and also for eczema, acne, and boils. Echinacea is also a digestion aid but today it is used largely as an immunity booster. There are plenty of teas available containing echinacea, but you can also easily grow echinacea yourself. Dig a tiny bit of the root up in the spring to make your own decoction. See page 38 for directions for preparing roots and page 17 for directions of how to make a decoction.

Eucalyptus *(eucalyptus spp.)*

Elcho Island is well populated with eucalyptus, particularly the ghost gum tree. Eucalyptus figures prominently in dreamings and the holistic health of various groups of Australian Aboriginal people, including the Yolngu people I came to know so well. The eucalyptus leaf is an antiseptic enjoyed all across the world. Certain groups of Australian

Aborigines have been brewing them to soothe coughs and colds for thousands of years. The essential oils are also antiseptic, and they provide antiviral actions as well. Tasmanian blue eucalyptus is used as an inhalant for tuberculosis and upper respiratory complaints. This oil can also be dispensed through the air using a pot of simmering water or an aromatherapy-dedicated vaporizer. Lemon and peppermint eucalyptus (*E. citriodora* and *E. dives*) are also useful in the treatment of asthma, colds, and fever; lemon eucalyptus is an antifungal. Peppermint eucalyptus is a pain reducer useful for flu.

To enjoy the healing medicine of eucalyptus, simply hang a bunch of it on the showerhead. Tie with hemp string to affix. Steaming hot water releases the essential oils contained in the eucalyptus leaf.

Flaxseed *(Linum usitatissimum)*

Another useful winter herb is flaxseed. Flaxseed boosts fiber intake and contains important phytonutrients. It is a natural source of fiber, trace vitamins, minerals, amino acids, omega-3, and lignins. Two tablespoons is the amount commonly used—this portion contains seventy calories. Look for organic flaxseed. Buy the seeds whole. Grind using a mortar and pestle or with a coffee grinder until fine. Store ground and whole seeds as well as the oil in the refrigerator. To use: sprinkle this onto salads or main dishes, or add to smoothies, juices, shakes, or a nutritious hot cereal like oatmeal. Take flaxseed oil orally, one teaspoon a day, or add to salad dressing. Brewing flaxseed tea makes a very effective remedy for irregularity. You can also try flaxseed added to yogurt or juice. I recommend daily use of flaxseed meal.

AN ABORIGINAL VISION OF THE SEASONS OF LIFE

Winter is one of those times when we reflect on the skies. Many of the stories we know so well in the West revolve around the winter sky; the story of the bright star that led the three wise men to Bethlehem to find the baby Jesus is one example. We sing carols about this star and wonder what it was and how it came to be. Further afield in Australia, among the Yolngu people to whom I dedicated this book, there is the story of quite a different star.

Before sharing the story, I must admit that while I, like most people, am fascinated by indigenous cultures, it is all but impossible for a person not raised in indigenous culture to comprehend the traditions, even though many of us are descendants of aboriginal people. During the 1990s, I did have the rare privilege of living within an Australian Aboriginal community along with my family. This place is called Galiwin'ku and it is on the Aboriginal-owned island of Elcho, located on the Top End of Australia's Northern Territory.

In order to truly exist within that community, you must be affiliated with the people, who are called Yolngu. Typically the Yolngu will adopt outsiders so they have a place within their cosmology; this was the case with us. My family and I were adopted and given aboriginal names, moieties (an elaborate network of clan affiliations), totemic animals, and an extended family, thereby we gained a place in their society.

Unfortunately, while we were there, someone died. As a member of that deceased person's clan, I was permitted to be "painted up" (painted with a local white clay and natural ochres) and to dance the secret women's business dances of our clan. We danced like the totemic animals affiliated with us—a type of turtle and the ibis that flourish on the island. This was my first time of seeing Morning Star. It has taken more than a decade for me to begin to understand this highly symbolic star.

Morning Star is part amulet and charm in much the same way as a mojo. It is also an exquisite sculpture. I say part amulet, charm, and sculpture, because it is a highly specialized traditional object with spiritual implications, painted with symbols that speak of the clan's dreaming, which is also visually alluring. People of the Dhuwa moiety use Morning Star poles during post-funerary ceremony. The stories and ritual connected with Morning Star symbolize the passage of the soul from one state of being to another—what we call a passage of life. Morning Star represents the inner spirit world before birth, the physical phase of life, death, and the life in the land of the ancestors.

Morning Star utilizes the analogy of going from dawn to dusk to describe our passage through life, and it reminds me of an emblem of spiritual winter. How it works is the ancestors keep Morning Star in a special bag, woven of ancient palm fronds and colored with natural dyes, called a dilly bag. The ancestors send the dilly bag containing the star out at night on a long string. It works like a fishing line—they toss it out as far as possible and then reel it in in the morning at sunrise.

Traditionally, the Yolngu people call it Banumbirr in their language. Banumbirr has feathers, symbolic of monsoonal rains, which bring the ibis and a time of fertility on its wings. The phallic shape of the pole itself symbolizes procreation. Morning Star symbolizes the ways the Sun moves in relation to the Earth and uses that activity to symbolize the cycle of life, our abiding relationship with the ancestors' and our place within the seasons.

Garlic *(Allium sativum)*

Those with chronic bronchitis and compromised immune systems can utilize raw garlic in salads, minced and sweetened with honey, or as a tea. For the hardy, eat garlic whole or mince and add to water; drink immediately. This gives a buzz of energy, which is quite nice when you are feeling worn down. Garlic is a digestive aid that clarifies the liver and gall bladder. Garlic is known to reduce blood pressure and help with circulatory problems. Garlic juice and supplements are used as an expectorant and to treat stomach flu.

Ginger *(Zingiber officinale)*

Ginger can be infused to make tea; serve hot or iced as a tea with lemon. Cooking with grated or dried ginger (adding ½–1 teaspoon depending on size of meal) adds zest and warmth to just about any dish. Ginger is warming and anticatarrhal, and can be used as a tonic, detoxifier, and digestive aid. It speeds elimination and lowers cholesterol and blood pressure.

Hyssop *(Hyssopus officinalis)*

Hyssop is a strong herb that is ideal for treating winter ailments. Hyssop helps with stomachache from holiday overeating and treats indigestion. It is good for general complaints including sore throat, breast and lung problems, cough, colds, nose and throat infection, mucus congestion, gas, and catarrh.

Hyssop should not be used for extended periods. Taking ½ to 1½ cups per day for three to four days per month should be the limit. To prepare, steep one teaspoon hyssop in ½ cup boiled water. Use hyssop sparingly.

Lemon *(Citrus limonum)*

Lemons are highly touted by the Gullah and Hoodoos. The Gullah use lemon in herbal teas as a natural remedy. Lemon is often combined with herbal tea and honey to treat the symptoms of cold or flu. It can also be paired with honey and taken by the spoonful for sore throat and coughs—the two enhance the efficacy of herbal teas when treating cold and flu. I suggest one teaspoon of your favorite honey mixed with ½ teaspoon lemon juice for sore throat—take as needed.

Life Everlasting *(Gnaphalium polycephalum)*

The bright yellow flowers of the life everlasting plant address body, mind, and spirit. Infuse the flowers in hot water to make a tonic that deters illness. Life everlasting tea with fresh lemon juice is a Gullah treatment for colds and a fever. Hoodoos place life everlasting inside mojo bags as a good health charm.

Mullein *(Verbascum thapsus)*

Mullein is a gentle treatment for coughs and colds, lung weakness, asthma, and bronchitis, and it is also calming and soothing to the lungs and bronchial tubes. It contains vitamins and flavonoids as well as saponins that cleanse the body. To create mullein tea, add one teaspoon of herb to one cup of boiled water. Strain. Flavor if desired with lemon and honey.

Onion *(Allium cepa)*

Onion is a relative of garlic (*Allium* spp.) and it is useful in much the same way. Use raw or juiced onion to treat cough or stomachaches, as a tonic, for antiseptic purposes, to reduce blood pressure, and to increase virility. Some people in the Caribbean grate onion and soak it in a cup of water, then sip the water all day to reduce weight. To enhance its efficacy and improve the taste, lemon and honey can be added to onion water to boost immunity. Add thinly sliced raw Vidalia onion to salads or sandwiches. Make it a habit to season your food using minced onion, as the first ingredient that you sauté. Sauté using virgin olive oil—this is tasty, heart-healthy, and it reduces the need for large amounts of salt.

Peppermint *(Mentha piperita)*

Peppermint was once considered a panacea—cure-all—for just about every known discomfort. Peppermint tea works as a decongestant when inhaled from a pot of simmering water. Just put a towel over your head to form a tent (be careful not to allow it to touch the flames) and inhale the aromatic peppermint. It will help clear the nasal passage and chest. Inhaling peppermint is also a treatment for both laryngitis and bronchitis. In England, peppermint tea is consumed to decrease the severity and length of colds at their onset. Putting a couple of tea bags inside a washcloth works as a compress to relieve headache and body pain associated with influenza. Its ability to reduce pain makes it useful also as a mouthwash for toothache, gum disease, and cavities. Peppermint also soothes the nerves and lifts mild depression, which can strike due to illness or light deprivation. Peppermint tea is made from the dried herb in the same way as mullein.

Rum

In her book *Jamaican Culture and International Folklore*, Jamaican author Claudette V. Copney shares a variety of herbal remedies featuring bay laurel leaf prepared as rum.

Flu

Rub down person with bay rum to draw out fever; stay under covers. During headache, pour bay rum on a small face cloth, inhale as needed.

Nose Bleeds

Soak cloth in bay rum, pin around head, and inhale vapors.

Tone Internal Organs (cure-all)

Add one shot of bay rum to coffee or tea any time of day.[1]

CHAPTER SEVEN

Elders

Ancestors, Dreaming, Remembrance, and Community Health

In African society and other indigenous cultures, community is of vital importance. At the center of community and family life is the elder. Elders are celebrated for their wisdom and are seen as reservoirs of information regarding families and the culture at large.

Interestingly enough, according to Celtic tradition, the Elder Moon appears just as it gets really cold, the time between Thanksgiving and Yule. Elder Moon marks the darkest days of the year; it asks us to remember our own mortality and our role in the cycle of life. For Wiccans, the elder tree is sacred. This tree leads the mind through the haze and confusion of life, guiding us through the spiral path that leads to the sacred ground where birth and death coexist.

As you reflect on the mystery of Elder Moon, it is also important to remember that winter is the time to stay in close communication with elders of the community. Elderly people suffer greatly from ailments that young people recover from quite easily, like colds and the flu. It is important to check in with family members who are seniors, and it is a very nice gesture to call on elderly neighbors.

In this chapter, there is a plethora of ideas for nurturing the health of the elder, from immunity boosters to foot soaks and massage. If you don't have time for these things, a simple cup of peppermint tea or ginger beverage would do a great deal to revitalize the spirits of your elders. This section features information and recipes geared toward the health of elders. Herbal massage, tonics, memory boosters, home spa, sleep aids, and a fun group project are included.

Elder Tree *(Sambucus nigra)*

The elder tree has much to offer seniors in the community as the tree symbolizes stability and wisdom. Infusion of elder flowers promotes perspiration and treats rheumatic complaints when used as an oil infusion, ointment, or salve. Elder flowers ease depression and serve as a relaxant and treatment for puffy eyes and rheumatism.

Elder Ritual

According to many indigenous belief systems, including those of the Celts, various groups of Native Americans, and in traditional African spirituality, trees should be asked to provide healing energy—it should never be assumed that healing energy is there to be taken. The tree should also be thanked when using any of its parts for herbal healing.

To begin this ritual, cup a handful of elder flowers firmly, and on the count of four, breathe in their dainty aroma while considering the potential you hold in your hands. In a smooth, controlled count of four, breathe out your wish for the flowers to release their healing ashe in the brew you are about to take. On your next inhalation, thank the tree for its flowers. Continue this meditation using a four-count for inhaling and a four-count for exhaling, as is common in Hatha Yoga pranayama (breathing meditation). If you regularly cultivate pranayama, feel free to extend the time between breaths, deepening to an eight-, ten-, or twelve-count rather than four. Focus only on your breath and the flowers. Repeat this until you are deeply relaxed and find yourself in a meditative though mindful state.

Steep one cup elder flowers in four cups hot water. Dip two cotton squares in elder tea, put in a bowl, then place it in the freezer. Strain one cup of infusion; set aside. Pour remaining tea with flowers into the basin. Have your elder put her feet up, relax, and drink tea (with honey and lemon if desired). Test temperature of elder infusion in the basin; when it is not too hot, add one teaspoon lavender buds. Have your elder place her feet into the floral infusion. Then put the cotton squares on her eyes. Let her relax as long as she'd like, then gently towel dry her feet and have a pair of comfortable slippers waiting to complete the spa.

Elder trees are imbued with many mysteries connected with death, resurrection, and rebirth. The glyph of elder means, "I am a wave of the sea." "On the boundless sea, I was set adrift." "All of these things shall pass away but the soul and spirit shall remain."

Dead Sea Salt

Salt, as the essence of the sea, is a wonderful substance, symbolic of life and an enhancement for our lives during the coldest days of winter. Dead Sea salt is a natural substance from Israel, used in a bath to encourage relaxation and reduce tension, body aches, and headaches. Salt is associated with spiritual cleansing, nurturance, and the Mothers of the Sea.

Epsom Salts

Epsom salt is recommended for relaxing strained or bruised muscles. The combination of Dead Sea and Epsom salts can help the winter spirit reach a relaxed state. Salts are believed to be rejuvenating to the over-worked body, mind, and spirit.

Sea Kelp, also called Bladderwrack (*Fucus visiculosus*)

Used magically in the following bath salt, sea kelp works with the spirits of the ocean and is a protective healing plant. Sea kelp encourages positive vibrations, psychic abilities, and prosperity. It also contains important vitamins and minerals for skin care.

Crone Wisdom Bath Salt

    2 cups Epsom salt
    2 cups coarse Dead Sea salt
    2 cups fine sea salt
    ½ cup sea kelp
    1 teaspoon each: chamomile and lavender essential oils

Put first three ingredients in bowl. Sprinkle with essential oils. Stir. Pour into a large glass or metal screw-top container. Add sea kelp. Shake.

Let rest forty-eight hours. Use one or two cups per bath. Soak for twenty minutes or more.

Yemaya-Ologun Bath Ritual

To the Yoruba people of Nigeria and other followers of Ifa, Yemaya-Ologun is an angelic deity that embodies the spirit of creation. This spirit lives in natural bodies of water. She is thought of as the Great Mother or Cosmic Womb. This powerful mother figure is beloved by many for her capacity for deep understanding and generosity. To invoke the spirit of Yemaya-Ologun, try this spirited bathroom ritual.

Create an altar on your bathroom window ledge, table, or tub as follows:

1. Clean the designated surface (ledge, table, or tub) by lightly brushing with a feather.

2. Lay down a white satin or white silk cloth.

3. Arrange cowrie and conch shells (or other available sea-shells) on the cloth.

4. Put a rock or fish fossil in the center of the shells.

5. Put a glass of vodka, brandy, or rum next to the circle of shells, and surround it with coins facing north, south, east, and west. This is your spirit glass.

6. Dip a crystal or semi-precious stone in the spirit glass and then set it on top of the central rock (or fossil).

7. Set out a few tropical leafy green plants or ferns.

8. Light frankincense or myrrh incense, burn tobacco or a blue candle.

9. Add bath salts under running water in the plugged bathtub.

10. Relax and enjoy!

Black Cocoa Butter Body Bliss Treatment

I love this silky treat for achy muscles around the back, shoulders, and wrist joint areas. You know, the type of pain we get from using the computer keyboard and gazing at the monitor a little too long? This treatment is simply delightful.

1. Warm up the sore area using one of these methods:

   › Fill a hot water bottle with very hot but not boiling water and seal tight—be careful not to scald yourself.

   › Warm a flax-filled body pillow in the microwave for the recommended amount of time. (Mitts for sore hands and booties for tired feet are widely available at health food stores, pharmacies, and spas.)

   › Apply a warm heating pad to the area.

2. Have your partner or a friend scoop out some of the cocoa butter and warm it by pressing his or her hands together until it is melted.

3. Remove heat source (selected from above).

Your partner can then apply the melted cocoa butter directly to the painful area, massaging until you feel your tight muscles released.

Arnica *(Arnica montana)*

Arnica is well respected as a treatment for pain, rheumatism, sore muscles, and joints. It is typically extracted in oil and used as a warming massage. (Please use caution as arnica has been known to cause allergic reactions such as dermatitis for some individuals.)

To make arnica oil, fill a sterile jar loosely with arnica flowers and cover with safflower, sweet almond, grape seed, or olive oil. Cap, then store away from direct sunlight for six to eight weeks. Swirl daily to release arnica into the oil.

Foraha, also called Tamanu *(Calophyllum inophyllum)*

Foraha is a dark green oil with a thick and waxy consistency. This oil has a wide array of medicinal qualities including its analgesic, anti-inflammatory, and antibiotic capabilities. Foraha is useful in the treatment of wounds, eczema, burns, insect bites, herpes, varicose veins, and scars. It makes a nutritious face oil. Revered for its ability to regenerate cell growth, foraha oil is also a treatment for fragile or broken capillaries. Foraha oil is great for massaging sore muscles and aching feet, legs, or joints. It has a strongly nutty smell, which can be counteracted by adding a few drops of lavender, clary sage, or sandalwood essential oil. A single drop of rose otto or neroli would also mask the nutty smell. Each of these essential oils conditions the skin and is generally relaxing as well.

Tonic Teas

Earlier in this chapter, numerous herbs were presented to calm, soothe, comfort, boost immunity, and fight illnesses. The following herbs are considered systemic tonics. They have been used historically to boost memory as well.

Ginkgo *(Ginkgo biloba)*

At two hundred million years old, ginkgo is the oldest tree in the world. Ginkgo leaves are associated with longevity and good health as well as memory. Ginkgo throat spray is used in Chinese medicine to reduce allergies. Ginkgo also facilitates good circulation. Proper circulation helps concentration, which in turn supports the function of memory. Ginkgo tea or extracts can also be used to reduce headache, maintain balance and equilibrium, reduce strokes, and assist with hearing.

Mugwort *(Artemsia vulgaris)*

Mugwort is associated with the elder wisdom of the crone. Mugwort is a hardy plant with feathery leaves that spreads quickly and can pop up anywhere. Mugwort is used in a bath to treat rheumatism, fatigue, and gout. This herb is harmful in high doses, and it should not be taken if you are pregnant.

To make mugwort tea, steep one teaspoon herb in half cup of water, and sip throughout the day. (Limit to half cup daily.)

Rosemary *(Rosmarinus officinalis)*

Like gingko, rosemary is a systemic tonic for the heart and mind. Rosemary is associated with love and remembrance. This herb helps blood circulate efficiently, facilitating concentration and helping memory. Rosemary relaxes nerves, though it is a tonic to the system. It contains a substance called rosmarinic acid, which has an antiviral and antimicrobial function in the body. Rosemary aids healing from upper respiratory ailments like bronchitis, and it generally speeds recovery from numerous complaints because of its high level of antioxidants. The tea also darkens gray hair when used as a rinse.

Sage *(Salvia officinalis)*

Sage has many of the same properties as rosemary. It has been highly regarded throughout history as a tonic, an aid to longevity, and a stimulant to the memory. This herb is useful to women going through menopause and those with fevers as it reduces perspiration. Sage tea soothes the nerves, curtails trembling, and eases mild depression.

Sage tea, like rosemary, can be applied to the hair as a darkening rinse. The two herbs darken hair slowly through a staining process, resulting from the tannins they contain.

To use: steep one teaspoon herb in half a cup of water. Limit use to one cup a day and then only use occasionally, not on a daily basis. Excessive use of sage is dangerous and potentially toxic. *It should not be taken if you are breastfeeding.*

Saint John's Wort *(Hypericum perforatum)*

Saint John's wort flowers are very helpful with body aches when extracted in oil. Follow the same directions as for arnica on page 93. Saint John's wort is also used as a tea for mild to moderate depression. (It can make skin sensitive to the sun if used frequently.)

Winter Dreaming

In some Native American cultures, the mid-winter festival is a time to share and examine the dreams of the community. During this important festival, dreams are collected, recorded, and celebrated. This is the time when one of the most feared animals in North America, the bear, sleeps. In many ways, the behavior of the bear reflects our own. She has stored up food and now draws on the energies of spring, summer, and fall to make it through winter. Mother bears give birth to their cubs during this time of the year, yet they do not fully realize this because they are in hibernation. The birth mimics the rebirth of our spirit. New life is something that we can appreciate fully in the spring. Bears are also connected with healing. They are thought to be capable of bridging the world of humans with that of the ancestral spirits.

Dream Pillow

Dream pillows, such as the one described here, deter insomnia and encourage fascinating dreams. This is designed as a group project for up to eight participants. If you are working on your own, store extra pillows in an airtight container or Ziploc bag until ready to use.

The following makes enough for eight dream pillows.

Dried lemon verbena leaves
Dried rose petals
Dried chamomile flowers
Dried French lavender buds
Dried bay
Dried mullein
Spanish moss
Dried hops
⅛ teaspoon chamomile essential oil
½ teaspoon French lavender essential oil
6 drops attar of roses (or ½ teaspoon rose fragrance oil)
2 teaspoons orrisroot, powdered

Crumble first six ingredients into a large bowl until fine. Tear Spanish moss into one-inch pieces. Add hops (an allergen, see below). Sprinkle essential oils over bruised herbs. Stir in orrisroot powder. Mature the mixture by placing it in a dark jar away from direct light. Shake daily for four to six weeks. While waiting for the mixture to mellow, each participant should make a small dream pillowcase using gingham, linen, hemp, or other fabric scraps. Use two nine-inch squares of fabric and cotton thread. This particular dream pillow is designed to encourage strength, restful deep sleep, and prophetic dreams when slipped inside a standard pillowcase.

Note: Allergy-sensitive individuals should wear a dust mask to complete this project.

Dream-Telling Circle

A dream pillow can be a powerful tool for observing mid-winter, particularly for seniors. Bring a small group of people together to make the pillows. A week or two later, meet again to discuss dreams inspired by them.

If this is not possible, have those around you write down their dreams and put them into a collective jar. The following year during mid-winter, have a special dinner and go through the dream jar, sharing and interpreting each other's dreams.

Examining dreams is an age-old way of storytelling, connecting with and remembering those who have passed beyond. Dream-telling is a strong African tradition that has survived to the present day.

Pleasant Dream Tea

Enjoy a good night's sleep using herbs and flowers. Select from the following dried herbs or any combination: jasmine flowers, hops, lavender, chamomile, catnip, peppermint, or valerian. Avoid hops if you are recovering from addictions; they act as a catalyst for some people.

Add two teaspoons of herb to strainer, set aside. Boil water. Pour one cup boiling water in the cup (without herbs). Heat cup three minutes; pour out water. Add strainer. Pour hot water over herbs—cover, steep ten minutes. Add honey and milk or lemon if desired.

Jamaican Hot Toddy

Warm one cup milk with one crushed cardamom pod; when milk is very hot, remove cardamom pod. Add one shot of Jamaican rum.

Death, Release, and Remembrance

Death becomes a reality during the winter. The landscape, colors, and even the temperature are all suggestive of death. Death has positive aspects. For example, decomposing matter becomes nourishing mulch for new plants, as I discussed earlier in the case of neem leaves. Death makes way for the birth of the new, physically and metaphysically if we consider the story of Jesus Christ. Each New Year, we celebrate the death of old times and old ways that have a negative effect on our lives. Death, as embodied by winter, offers a chance for renewal, growth, and change. Even inclement weather, the phenomena that we dread and curse, plays an important role, as it gives us no choice but to slow down, pause, and think about our lives.

For those of us who have lost people who are dear, death can be a harsh reality. Elders keenly feel this relationship with death, as often their friends and loved ones have passed on. The following incense is made with a combination of herbs with magical qualities designed to address all the issues that winter stirs:

Release Incense

5 bay leaves
3 anise stars
2 small cinnamon sticks or ¼ cup cinnamon chips
Handful uva ursi, mint leaves, rosemary, and chamomile (dried)
3 myrrh chunks
7 frankincense tears
⅛ teaspoon each: myrrh, bay, and ylang ylang essential oils
Aquamarine and tourmaline (stone or bead)

Using a mortar and pestle or coffee grinder, pulverize bay, anise, and cinnamon until you have a coarse powder. Add to a bowl. Pulverize uva ursi, mint, rosemary, and chamomile using a mortar and pestle to release their essential oils. Add to the bowl. Grind myrrh and frankincense and add them to the bowl. Stir. Sprinkle essential oils over all ingredients. Mix. Place mixture and stones into a capped container. Shake daily for one week.

To use: burn release incense in a large seashell or on top of a stone; sprinkle a pinch of the incense on a hot charcoal. Replace as needed. Release grief, sorrow, despair, or communications to the spirits into the smoke.

Remembrance Garland

Garlands are an age-old symbol of winter that captures the magic of the seasons. To create a remembrance garland, string pieces of cockscomb, bay leaves, cranberries, orange peels, dried lemon slices, cinnamon stick, and allspice. Soak cranberries, cinnamon, allspice, bay, and orange in Florida water or Kananga water (substitute plain water if specialty waters are unavailable). The next day, cut a suitable length of waxed linen or hemp string for the welcoming area of your home. Begin the strand and end it with cranberries, create your own pattern with remaining botanicals. Remembrance garland is a fragrant invitation for your ancestors and departed loved ones.

Spring

CHAPTER EIGHT

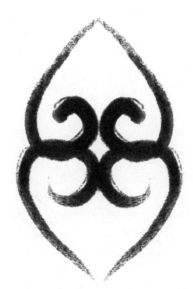

Spring into Ritual

Rain, Thunder, Water Element, and Flowers

Spring Equinox Ritual and Ceremony: Welcoming Spring with the Goddesses

The spring is called variously Ostara, the vernal equinox, and the spring equinox. Spring is that special time of the year focused on awakening, new beginnings, growth, development, and balance. For many, spring stirs new feelings to life.

Forced Bulbs

Nature has its own rhythm—we know it and should respect it. Sometimes, especially during winter, we long for the blossoms of spring, wanting the sweet breath of Mother Nature to grace our homes. Bulb forcing provides an opportunity to bring heavenly scents and pleasing colors into your home. Today there is a renewed sense of pleasure in the hobby, hence all of the available bulb forcing kits. You can "force" a bulb to bloom early by simulating the conditions in nature that encourage bulbs to bloom each spring through the fall.

Hardy bulbs work best for this project, for example: crocus (*Crocus* sp.), daffodils (*Narcissus* sp.), hyacinths (*Hyacinthus* spp.), and tulips (*Tulipa* spp.). Less commonly forced but still workable bulbs include

Dutch iris (*Iris x hollandica*), snowdrop (*Galanthus* sp.), grape hyacinth (*Muscari* spp.), and Star-of-Bethlehem (*Ornithogalum* spp.).

Forcing bulbs requires: (1) planning (begin late summer to early fall for Yule or other winter holiday blossoms), (2) selection of desired bulbs, (3) planting, (4) cooling, and (5) forcing bulbs to flower.

This is another wonderful family project. I've noticed young children are especially fond of growing their own plants. To begin this project, select bulbs and an appropriate pot or pots. Next prepare a well-drained potting soil. Mix equal parts of indoor potting soil, sphagnum peat moss (great for aerating), and Perlite for good drainage. After you mix this, add it to a clean pot that has a hole at the bottom for drainage.

If you use clay pots, soak them overnight. This helps the potted bulbs stay moist.

Bulbs will differ in how deeply they should be planted, but it is at the same depth for each species as you would use in the outdoor garden. For a rule of thumb, the very large bulbs (tulip and daffodil types) should be loosely covered with the top of the bulb uncovered; small bulbs (crocus, snowdrops, and grape hyacinth) are completely covered with the potting mix. Water.

To cool, expose the bulbs to an unheated area of the home if available, like an unfinished basement or crawl space, or set outside if it is between 35 and 50 degrees Fahrenheit. Cool for three to four months.

After the cooling period, bring the bulbs to a place indoors that is fairly warm (60 to 65 degrees Fahrenheit). Place them in a shady location, water, and keep soil moist. When shoots appear, bring the bulbs into the regular living area with warmer temperatures (about 70 degrees) and natural sunlight. Make sure all sides of the plant receive even light by rotating the pot periodically. With care, you will have flowers in three to four weeks.

Note: Narcissus and amaryllis (*Hippeastrum cultivars*) are usually forced much more easily and quickly than other bulbs, without the extensive cooling period. You'll find these in your home and garden center, through your florist, or sometimes in the supermarket already planted in soil and ready to take home and water. Typically these types are begun in the late fall around Thanksgiving and will produce blooms between Yule and New Year.

Naturally Colored Eggs

Eggs are used in prosperity, abundance, crossroads, and fertility rites as they are associated with spring. There are many natural dyes available, and they enhance the magical nature of eggs. I encourage experimentation with natural teas to enhance the natural beauty inherent in the promise of eggs.

Tea-Stained Crackled Eggs

I recommend making tea-stained crackled eggs as follows:

> 3 tea bags (rose hips yield a soft red, currant and blueberry
>   yield soft purples, and black tea makes tan)
> 24 ounces water
> 6 eggs

Put the eggs in sixteen ounces of cold water in a pot. Set heat at medium-high. Boil twenty minutes. Put one cup of the water in a separate kettle. Make tea. Let steep fifteen minutes. Tap each egg lightly to crack the surface. Put the eggs in a bowl with the tea. Soak overnight. In the morning, remove—blot excess tea, display as desired.

Isis Snake Divination

Spring is the time of nature revelation and discovery. Just as plants peek out of the ground, so do snakes and other creatures that have rested over the winter. March is the time of Isis, moon mother and mother of the sea. Snakes are one of her symbols. This ritual respectfully conjures her symbolic reptile, paying tribute to her while invoking her spirit.

1. Draw a bath.

2. Add ¼ cup Epsom salt, ¼ cup coarse and ¼ cup fine Dead Sea salt.

3. Put on a piece of moonstone (ring, necklace, bracelet, or anklet).

4. Light a blue candle, place on a fireproof container near the bathtub.

5. Bring a crystal ball with you into the bath.

6. Gaze at the candle as you breathe deeply and very slowly until you are very relaxed. Realize that you are bathing in the smoke of Isis.

7. Call her name quietly but deliberately, drawing it out slowly like a snake's hiss, "I-sis, I-sis, I-sis." Breathe in and with the exhale whisper "I-sis" for about five minutes.

8. Lift the crystal ball into the air once you feel the spirit of Isis within the room. Hold the ball in front of the candle flame. See what is in store as you divine by scrying both fire and crystal.

Mujaji: the Rain Goddesses

Here is a group of goddesses believed to have come to the earth in the opposite region of Africa from the Isis homeland, South Africa. Goddesses seem mythic, divine, often outside of the realm of mere mortals; yet in parts of southeastern Africa, there is the belief that certain rain goddesses came down to earth to inhabit the bodies of queens. This segment explores the *Mujajis*, the goddess queens whose lineage continues to the present day. Before we get to our work, here is a snapshot of the Mujajis' background and beginnings. It's always best to have some understanding of a goddess before invoking her energy.

A Mujaji is a goddess in the flesh, a sacred leader of the Shona. Shona are people from southern Africa who speak a Bantu-based language called ChiShona and live in the areas in and around Lovedu. The Mujaji ("Transformer of the Clouds") is the goddess of fertility, sustenance, cycles, and life itself, and she hails from a distinctive line of rain-makers beginning with Mambo Monomotapa. Mujaji I is the first of these goddesses. She came to live on earth around 1800 CE. Mugede, the last in a line of mortal male rulers, fathered Mujaji I at the end of his reign in 1800, and later he fathered Mujaji II. As a result of the inces-tuous relationship, the second rain queen was both daughter and half sister to Mujaji I, and so it has gone for many generations.

During the leadership of the males ending with Mugede, there was strife, aggression, war, and social unrest. Near the end of his reign, Mugede received a divine message that the leadership of his nation should turn strictly female. Females in the Lovedu society associate women rulers with order, peace, prosperity, nurturing, and appeasement.

The Mujajis' exploits are legendary, and most of their society is related to them through arranged marriages. The Zulu regard them as the great magicians of the north because they seem to control every-thing from weather to the day-to-day goings-on of the community. Mujaji I produced copious rain during the first half of the 20th century. Leaders including Soshanganga of Gazaland, Shaka of the Zulu, and Mosweshwe of the Sotho appealed to Mujaji I for rain. During numer-ous African wars, Mujaji had a reputation for producing rain, provid-ing sustenance, washing out inroads and deterring invaders, saving her people repeatedly.

Mujaji is immortal and relatively inaccessible. She is at the center of life, as only she possesses the power to create rain, change seasons, or inflict society with droughts or floods. If she is angry or upset, there is no rain and this leads to horrendous droughts. This is why she is also called "Queen of the Locusts" and "Queen of Drought," as well as a four-breasted marvel. Their temperamental quality is another reason why the rain queens are greatly feared. Constant care, respect, and vigi-lance to their honor are required year 'round to ensure their continuous assistance. The Mujaji rain queens continue to be with us through myth and legend. Their contemporary descendants have no military power but still yield spiritual influence within their community because of their ability to conjure rain. With the major seasons in Africa being the wet and the dry, there is a great deal of emphasis on conjuring life-sustaining rain in dry times. John Anenechukwu Umeh, whom I men-tioned in chapter one, offers another rare glimpse into the magical uses of the element water by West Africa's Igbo people with the following three examples:

> Igba ogogo mmili is "dancing waters," since ogogo is an excitedly playful washing of one's body during a rain shower, without collecting the rain into any vessel or container.

> Mmili uji osisi is water gathered from natural bowls or depressions or holes in trees.

> Mmili akwukwo osisi is water gathered by plant and tree leaves.[1]

Collecting the Essence of Mujaji

Try some of these Igbo methods of interacting with the rain when you feel that your ideas are stale and lack creativity. Of course, those of you desiring physical fertility to bear children can also benefit from this engagement. To do your own *Igba ogogo mmili* bath, take a wash outdoors during a rain shower, nude if possible. Try gathering water from inside burls and other depressions in the surfaces of trees.

Get into the Water

Instead of hiding out from rain, sulking, or complaining about it, shift your focus to the gift of rain. Without rain, life as we know it would most likely cease to exist. Get into rain, literally. Here are some ways to enjoy the rain and use it in your life:

> Rainwater is easy to collect on the ground. Collection from a rural environment is best. Avoid collection sites near heavy traffic and do not collect rainwater from under eaves. Place multiple containers outside for greater quantity. Fresh rainwater is best but you can store rainwater in the fridge for a few days if necessary.

> Lightning water is collected from a thunderstorm. Lightning water is believed to bring dramatic changes to situations and can also bring an air of spontaneity or even capriciousness. Lightning water is associated with Yoruban orishas Shango and Oya.

> Use rainwater to bless your besom before spiritual cleansing, clearings, during the creation of a circle, or to bless a new grimoire.

> Use rainwater to charge or renew crystals, rocks, and minerals. Once they are cleansed, clear stones again with sun and moonlight.

> Record the sounds of rain or a thunderstorm. Play music during rites or ceremonies involving new beginnings, to generate ideas, to relax or meditate. High quality natural sound CDs or cassettes can also be purchased.

Essence of Hara Ke

This elixir continues to engage the spirit of the rain goddesses. This is a type of potpourri I use to bless my home and that of others under the inspiration of gods and goddesses. Since Hara Ke is one of the African rain goddesses, choose a rainy day of early spring to create her floral essence potpourri. This is designed to promote creativity, new beginnings, and fertility. Reflect on the revelation of one of these three facets of rain. Choose the one you desire the most in your home. Focus with great intention as you craft this blend.

4 cups dried pink rose petals mixed with whole dried rose buds
2 cups blue lavender
½ cup cut and sifted lemongrass
½ cup pine needles
1 cup dried lime slices
5-6 dried pomegranates
1 cup dried orange slices
⅛ teaspoon neroli
⅛ teaspoon jasmine absolute
⅛ teaspoon tuberose absolute
⅛ teaspoon attar of roses
¼ teaspoon eucalyptus essential oil
¼ teaspoon patchouli
⅛ teaspoon vetiver

½ teaspoon sandalwood oil

½ cup Queen Elizabeth root (pulverized) powder

5 cardamom pods ground

2 ground nutmegs

4 tablespoons ground cinnamon stick

Put first seven ingredients into a very large container, such as an extra-large mixing bowl or stockpot. Mix all of the absolutes and oils in a nonreactive bowl such as a Pyrex or stainless steel bowl. Blend oils with a stirring rod if you have one, or swirl. Take a moment to inhale this complex blend of scents, and listen to the rain as you focus on your intentions. Mix the four spices together in a separate mixing bowl. Pour the oils over the botanical blend. Mix. Shake on the powdered spices mix. Stir all together. Put in a plastic container with an airtight lid. Let mature for four to six weeks away from the direct sunlight and then it will be ready to use. Try the following ritual once it is mature.

Hara Ke Ritual

I remember seeing my godmother mist the tips of her broom with hydrosols like rose or lavender waters. You may have observed your elders doing this as well. It is always wise to observe the elders because many of their daily rites continue to have practical applications. The one I saw aids home cleaning with a broom since the wet bristles hold dust more readily than dry bristles. I also realize that natural water, fresh from a rain or thunderstorm, has a power all its own. You can refresh the energy in the home through judicious use of this type of natural force.

1. Take your special broom outside and tilt it upward so rain-drops wet the broom's bristles from the top.

2. Keep broom or besom upright until you get to the area you intend to ritualistically sweep. Sweep the bathroom floor with the rainwater-kissed broom. When you are finished, toss small bits of Essence of Hara Ke into bathtub and under throw rugs. By placing the essence under rugs, footsteps

release the energy, allowing you to engage in foot track magic of the Hoodoo.

3. As an auxiliary step, put a small closed jar of Essence Hara Ke near the bathtub. Open the jar while enjoying a soothing bath.

Pull energy down from the heavens, like rain pelting the thirsty Earth Mother—so shall you be replenished. Close the jar after the ritual.

Rain Season Ceremony

Here is a third way to work the rain:

1. Bring a floating candleholder outdoors on an evening of heavy rains during the new or waning moon.

2. Leave this out overnight in a safe location.

3. Go outside at dusk the next evening wearing all white. (If it is still raining, bring the candle bowl inside to conduct ritual).

4. Focus on your intentions then place three small, lit, white or pink floating flower candles inside bowl of rainwater using your dominant hand.

5. Face west. Recite as you continue to focus on the floating candles:

As rain comes from the sky

Show me the reasons to try

Drops of the rain goddesses, fresh as morning dew

Cleanse, renew

Sweet Mujaji, make everything in my sight

Bright, fresh, and sparkling like you

Recite this three times building intensity with each invocation.

6. Gaze at the fire as you visualize a successful transformation.

7. Use some of the rainwater on your fingers to snuff each candle.

8. Lift your hands high in the air. As the smoke is released toward the night sky chant,

    So it is written, so it will be done!

9. Gently blow the smoke so that it will carry your messages forward.

Like the rain from above, let your energy, passion, and creativity flow.

Remember to look forward to rain, welcome it, and use it in your magical workings.

Thank the Mujaji goddesses of the rain daily for the gifts they bestow upon the earth.

Thunder Orisha Invocation

Whereas we can have a tendency to shrink away from rain, thunder invokes fear. In Ifa, there is an important orisha and cult dedicated to working thunder. Shango is the magnetic warrior deity with a large personality. His tremendous inner energy force raises thunder. He is noble, elegant, protective, and tricky. To engage the positive aspects of this deity, go outside where there are plenty of trees—his element.

1. Face northeast, as it is his direction.

2. Burn his favorite incense, frankincense tears, in a censer, careful to use fireproof protective surfaces.

3. Spread cayenne peppers, hibiscus flowers, and bay leaves around the circumference of a tree that has some of Shango's characteristics.

4. Keep your head low; defer to this spirit.

5. Walk away backward, as quickly as possible without falling, until you are well away from the tree.

First Week of April

Seed Moon Abundance Ritual

Now that you have engaged the rain and thunder, don't forget about the area's wildlife; this is vital year-round. Just about any place you live will have birds. Birds are magical and they also have needs like all the earth's creatures. Together you can assist one another. The spell works like a charm. Celebrate Seed Moon by planting seeds of positive energy for greater abundance.

1. Go out under the light of Seed Moon, dig a shallow hole, then bury all of your pocket change.

2. Draw a symbol of love or peace out of wild birdseed.

3. Leave them out for forty-eight hours.

4. At the end of this period, most of your seed and the symbol will be consumed and spread elsewhere, bringing your wish for peace and love along with the seed. In the morning, plant a few sunflower seeds on this spot. During the growing season, birds and butterflies will continue to grow and spread your message of love and peace.

A year later, your abundance of change should flow back your way. Look for your change—most likely it will have doubled.

Spring Break Traveler's Spell

When I was growing up, people seldom took spring breaks. Today, it is something of a college student's rite of passage to travel someplace warm during the spring. Many young families find it a convenient time to get away to places like Disneyland. Others find ways to take advantage of this break from school and work schedules by doing fun projects at home or in their community. If your journey crosses water, try this helpful spell for a bon voyage.

On the day of Mercury (Wednesday), during the waxing cycle of the moon, it is the time to undertake a spell dedicated to successful travel by engaging the herb of seafarers, Irish moss. Irish moss ensures prosperity and abundance in all of your work. Gratefully use dried Irish moss, knowing that it comes from the depths of our sea mothers.

1. Crumble it finely over a bowl. Think: *safe by day, full at night*— repeat as a mental mantra.

2. Set the bowl out under the moonlight overnight.

3. Afterward, tuck some of this into your suitcase, a piece in each shoe.

4. Each night, visualize waves of prosperity rolling toward you from the sea. Hold the thought steadily, think of it frequently. Prosperity shall be yours!

CHAPTER NINE

Holistic Home

Spring Cleaning Mind, Body, and Spirit

Spring Tonic: Inner and Outer Beauty

Now here is something you don't see every day: a tonic that revitalizes energy and perks up weather-beaten hair—all in one. This spring tonic enhances hair color, brings gray from dingy to golden—and does the same for your spirit. It also brings depth to dark brown and black hair, lifts mood, relaxes anxiety, serves as an internal cleanser or a uterine tonic, gently stabilizes hormonal upsets, and boosts immunity. It contains equal amounts of oat straw, pau d'arco, black tea, lavender, bay leaves, parsley, chickweed, calendula, rosemary, sage, and marshmallow root.

To color hair: Add two tablespoons of the mixture to four cups of water. Bring to a boil.

Cover. Reduce heat to low. Infuse twenty minutes. Let cool. Strain well.

Just in Time for Mother's Day: Neroli Loofah Soap

The soft nature of neroli lends itself to the creation of your own hand-made soap. As a first step into soapmaking, purchase ready-made blocks of unscented soap called Melt and Pour (MP). These soap blocks, sold by the pound, are prepared using a variety of ingredients—some contain aloe vera, olive oil, shea butter, hemp, honey, or even oatmeal. Follow manufacturer's directions. If you enjoy color, add orange soap chips or even an orange Crayola crayon in the last stages of melting soap. Add the recommended amount of essential oil (neroli). You can enhance the orange scent further by adding three tablespoons of neroli hydrosol (orange blossom water) during the melting stage.

As a neat alternative, pour melted, scented soap over loofah sponges cut into one-inch slices and placed in a metal or Pyrex baking dish. Loofah sponge is a vegetable skeleton with unique exfoliating qualities. Most recipes create at least a dozen 3 x 5-inch blocks of soap—consider giving some away. Orange blossom soap makes a great gift for Mother's Day and only takes a few hours to complete. Wrap in clear wrapping paper and seal with a festive ribbon.

NATURAL DYES USING THE CATCH METHOD

The *catch method* is a way of infusing hair with natural dyes using repeated applications. Place a large bowl in a sink or bathtub. Lean over the bowl and then pour herbal rinse over your hair from a pitcher. Squeeze the rinse into the bowl. Pour liquid into pitcher. Repeat application ten to twelve times.

If dryness is a problem, you can add a teaspoon of warmed molasses, honey, or vegetable glycerin to the brew before using. Hot oil treatments with herbal oil, safflower oil, or melted shea butter might also be useful. The formula is designed to aid with hair growth, increase hair tensile strength, deter dandruff, add body, and soften and enhance color.

As an internal tonic, use one tablespoon herbs to one cup of water. Drink one to three times only, preferably in the evening, as it can be very relaxing and may cause a slight drowsy sensation. Add honey, fructose, or another sweetener if desired, with lemon or milk. It is designed to encourage internal flushing so be prepared!

As with all herbal preparations, this is excellent as a facial steam or hair steam. While preparing the brew, you can put your head and/or face over the pot using a hand towel as a tent to hold in steam. You should be very aware of flames and stay attentive in order to avoid burns or other fire hazards.

Finally, while this is an all-natural formula, presenting Mother Nature's best, if you should suffer allergic reactions, discontinue use. In rare instances, you could develop a rash. If this happens, rinse immediately with vinegar and water (one tablespoon to one cup). You could try the tonic again using a more diluted formula (add more water, use less herbs). Remember though, that this is only a courtesy warning. None of the ingredients used are known allergens if used as directed.

Stay Away Pest Mojo

A pleasurable spring cleaning activity is to put away the darker-colored heavy woolens and dense cottons of winter to make way for the lighter silks and linens of spring and summer. Once my clothing is clean and folded, I put it away until fall, and I'm sure many of you do the same. Try including this sachet mojo. Tucked into the closet, the bag is designed to keep insects away that might otherwise bore holes into some of your favorite sweaters. Here is the blend I craft for my entire family:

4 cups dried cedarwood chips
2 cups dried lavender buds
1 cup dried peppermint leaves
2 teaspoons cedarwood oil
2 teaspoons lavender essential oil
2 teaspoons pennyroyal essential oil
1½ teaspoon eucalyptus essential oil
1 teaspoon peppermint essential oil
½ teaspoon patchouli essential oil
½ teaspoon cassia essential oil

Pour cedarwood into a large bowl or stainless steel stockpot. Bruise lavender and peppermint by hand or with mortar and pestle. Crumbling these herbs releases their essential oils. In a separate small bowl, add essential oils one at a time. Swirl or mix with a stirring wand. Pour this over the herbs. Stir with a stainless steel spoon. Put this in an airtight container. Let it mature for four to six weeks. Put the blend into small muslin drawstring bags. Hang them in closets or on hangers, or put them in drawers or storage containers with fall and winter clothing. When you need these clothes again, they will smell clean and maintain their fresh appearance, especially if stored in bins or drawers.

Herbal Home Cleansing: Native American Smudging

Ancient Egyptians used a smoldering technique called *profomo* to clean and heal internal wounds with indigenous and imported resins and herbs. In the United States, one of the most influential incense cleaning methods is called smudging, designed by the Native Americans. Smudging goes well beyond dirt and grime. It is a type of holistic herbal cleansing addressing the spiritual, emotional, and physical aspects of clutter. While many people use sage almost exclusively for smudging, this segment shares some of our other lovely aromatic indigenous herbs, presented in the interest of plant sustainability. The incense herbs discussed are widely available and many are easily wildcrafted from your own property.

Opening the Way with a Sweetgrass Ritual
Sweetgrass (*Hierochloe odorata*) is often used at the beginning of rituals and ceremonies, as it is an invitation to positive nature spirits and the ancestors. A fragrant herb reminiscent of warmed vanilla, sweetgrass is sometimes called vanilla grass. It is beloved by various First Nation peoples, particularly the Sioux and Aniyunwiya or Tsalagi (commonly called Cherokee in English). The Lakota people connect this scented rush with the compassionate creation goddess Wohpe.

Wohpe is a striking, well-balanced, spiritual goddess associated with the mysterious seventh direction. She is thought to appear at the moment a puff of smoke appears. According to Lakota stories, the braided grasses symbolize the beautiful plaited hair of Wohpe though other nations associate sweetgrass with various other creation mothers.

Sweetgrass herb creates a quiet, seductive incense that assists during the process of spiritual cleansing, clearings, rituals, and blessings.

Like many beloved plants, sweetgrass is growing endangered in certain states, especially in some states along the East Coast and in New England. Sweetgrass grows in both North America and in Europe around the Arctic circle. In fact, the sacred nature of sweetgrass is shared among Native Americans and European groups who have utilized it as a strewing herb on church stairs during saint's days. Sweetgrass of different species is utilized to make the traditional baskets of the Gullah people as well. Truly a multicultural herb, sweetgrass has been cultivated for at least ten thousand years. Thirty species have been identified. Since the species *Hierochloe odorata* is disappearing rapidly, it is worth considering using the slightly less fragrant *H. alpina, H. hirta, H. occidentalis,* or *H. pauciflora.* Sweetgrass can also be cultivated and some people even grow it as an indoor houseplant under the right conditions.

Burning sweetgrass in the home is a simple yet evocative way to reconnect to the earth in accord with the advent of spring. Cultures across North America burn braided aromatic grass and rushes, not only sweetgrass but also whatever is fragrant and available locally. The smoldering grasses become a spiritual invitation for a fertile, vibrant spring with abundant rains that guarantee a safe harvest. Moreover, sweetgrass is noted for its antiseptic qualities. Create your own spring sweetgrass (or other aromatic wild grass) clearing ritual based on the following directions.

1. Cut wild aromatic grasses, or sweetgrass if available in your area, to about forty inches. Braid loosely in three strands. As an alternative, obtain a braid of sweetgrass from a reputable supplier.

2. Stroke the grass gently, and after that, whisper your wishes for the spring season.

3. Treat the sweetgrass as though it is the actual braid of Wohpe or another creation mother goddess.

4. Light the braid in a dark room, and implore the earth to open the way for you and your family to have an enlightened and abundant spring.

5. Tamp the flame and travel through your home, clockwise, in the four cardinal directions (east, south, west, and finally north) spreading her delightful vanilla scent and inherent wisdom along the way.

6. Focus on encouraging the positive vibrations from the smoke to bless your home as you travel carrying the braid.

Indigenous North American Incense Herbs

1. **Balsam fir** (*Abies balsamea*): Seneca blessings incorporate these sacred plants of the northern woodlands. Fir, popularly known as a "Christmas tree," has pleasing, aromatic qualities that are considered cleansing and purifying. Native to the northeastern United States and Canada, the Algonquin, Woodlands Cree, Iroquois, Menominee, Micmac, Ojibwa, and Potawatomi use balsam fir medicinally. The Ojibwa inhale the smoke from the needles to treat symptoms of a cold.

2. **Bayberry** (*Myrica pensylvanica*): This herb emits a pleasant fragrance when dried and burned as incense.

3. **Bearberry willow** (*Salix uva-ursi*): are prominent Native American healing trees.

4. **Bee Balm** (*Monarda didyma* and *Monarda* spp.): When bee balm is dried and used in incense blends, it has a fragrance reminiscent of oranges and mint combined.

5. **Cedar** (*Libocedrus decurrens, Juniperus monosperma*): Desert white cedar and California incense cedar are the preferred smudging cedars. Cedar is burned for a variety of reasons including prayer, invocation, and home blessings (for moving into a new home). The tree is believed to ward off

illness in the lodge and individuals, so it is used as smudging incense. Cedar works as a purifier and attraction herb when the woodchips are sprinkled over a hot charcoal block (see mesquite). **White Cedar** (*Thuja occidentalis*) is used by the Ojibwa and Potawatomi people, burned as incense in purification ceremonies.

6. **Cedarwood** (*Cedrus atlantica*): Wood chips can be used as a kindling source for other leaves and branches. Cedarwood is revered for its calming, balancing, ancient wisdom, and is considered a protective plant that aids focus while bringing clarity. The physical aspects are perfect for spring smudging blends; cedarwood is antiseptic and energizing.

7. **Juniper** (*Juniperus communis*): Juniper is a revered tree whose needles, berries, and wood are all useful in smudging blends. Juniper is celebrated because it is a tree that is uplifting, protective, and purifying, and also for its ability to boost confidence and energy levels. The physical uses include antiseptics, diuretics, and tonics. Southwestern groups have used juniper to ward off illness and ill intent.

8. **Mesquite** (*Prosopis glandulosa*): is a fragrant wood that is an ideal charcoal base for burning smoldering herbs during smudging.

9. **Mugwort** (see sagebrush).

10. **Pine** (*Pinus silvestris*): Pines are associated with endurance, perseverance, focus, trust, and stability. Healers celebrate the pine tree for its anti-infectious, antiseptic, tonic, stimulant, and restorative abilities. Pinyon pine needles are used by Southwestern groups such as the Navajo, Apache, Pueblo, and Zuni in smudging rites, sometimes in place of sweetgrass.

11. **Red willow** (*Salix lasiandra*): Also called osiers or Pacific willow, it grows in the western United States. Willows are prized in many tribes and used in ceremony for healing.

The Hidatsa people, whose name means "willow," are noted healers concentrated around the Missouri River. They have developed many medicinal uses for willow.

12. **Sagebrush** (*Artemisia tridenta* and *Artemisia* spp.): Wild sage is preferred over culinary sage (*Salvia officinalis* or *S. apiana*) as a smudging herb. Western Native American groups use sagebrush traditionally to treat colds. Sage is also considered protective of the spirit. It is also known to have antiseptic and tonic qualities to aid our energy levels. Sage is a very popular smudging herb, but **American sage** (*Salvia divinorum*) is a slow growing plant indigenous to a small area of the southwestern United States. Some types of sage, particularly American sage, are rapidly becoming endangered species because of their ever-increasing popularity as smudging herbs. Thus, it is important to use alternatives when possible, or to grow and cultivate the herb in your garden. **Mugwort** (*Artemisia vulgaris*) is a very useful, easy-to-grow alternative to the above listed sage genii, and is conducive to burning as smudging incense.

13. **White Spruce** (*Abies alba*): is considered a protective, renewing, grounding, and harmonizing tree that enables us to regain focus and clarity. Other healing properties include antidepressant, antiseptic, and stimulant actions.

In addition to these traditional native herbs, many people use lavender, hyssop, and rosemary because they are also holy plants that are widely available, easy to grow, and very fragrant.

The following directions offer guidance to help create your own smudge stick. Try to use home-grown plants or sprigs from trees on your property, bearing in mind that a part of the spirituality of using smudging herbs is that the herbs should not be bought or sold but traded, bartered, or harvested respectfully on your own, thanking the plant for each part taken. If you do not have any trees or herbs available, you might try bartering with a family member or friend.

1. Gather available sprigs and branches in the morning after dew has evaporated.

2. Cut each herb between twelve and eighteen inches.

3. Bundle the herbs, and then tie with hemp string.

4. Bring the bundle inside and hang it upside down away from direct sunlight.

5. Dry for several days—the bundle should still be pliable.

6. Lay the bundle on a natural fiber cloth or newspaper.

7. Fold, then roll the bundle until there is a neat six- to eight-inch-long bunch.

8. Bundle using natural hemp string or natural (undyed) cotton string.

Open a door or some windows for good ventilation and light a smudge stick. Tamp out the flame. Carry the smoking wand clockwise through each room of the home, emphasizing the four directions of the Medicine Wheel (east, south, west, and north—see side-bar "Smudging by the Crossroads"). Be attentive to all areas, smudging corners and crevices. Be especially attentive to areas that need cleansing or where unfortunate occurrences and arguments have taken place. Some people enjoy using a found bird feather to spread the smoke as they travel but your cupped hands are just as effective. This same approach could be used to help purify a new home, a nursery, or even a sickroom. Another style is achieved by crumbling an assortment of aloeswood, cedarwood, cinnamon bark, eucalyptus, juniper, pine, cedar, apple, or balsam poplar and burning it over a mesquite charcoal block, pieces of cedarwood, pinyon, or other fragrant wood.

Once you are finished with the cleansing ritual, dampen the smudge stick in seawater or rainwater. Hang it up to dry until the next time.

SMUDGING BY THE CROSSROADS

Many people enjoy a structure, so rather than leaving you to go willy-nilly with your smudging, here is a ritual you can follow if you desire. The Native American Medicine Wheel is similar to the Yowa Cross of the Yoruba cosmology, which we have adapted to a focus on crossroads—the mystical "X" shape. Visualize a crossroads. Go the center of the crossroads, as this is the seat of power. Relax; take cleansing breaths as you collect your energy and focus intention. Continue to do this as you visualize the four cardinal directions your movements will follow during smudging and clearing rituals. Begin to move to the east because that is where life begins—it is the place of birth and new beginnings. Travel next to the south, this is the place of the teenage years. West is next, for it represents midlife. End to the north, the place of the elder, wisdom, spirits, ancestors, and the afterlife. When smudging people, start with the heart, travel upward to the head. Next smudge the arms, and finally the legs and feet.

Traditional Cherokee people hang a braid of sweetgrass over each doorway inside the house for protection and as an invitation to positive spirits.

The positive aspects can be accentuated by adding other herbs such as pine or cedar branches. Some people with chronic upper respiratory disorders, babies, or elders may prefer having sweetgrass as living incense rather than burning it. This is accomplished by growing the plant in the home or garden or hanging as previously described.

Additional Uses for Smudging Herbs

Some people find smoke in the home disagreeable even with good ventilation. These are some alternate ways to use smudging herbs in the home.

1. The Sioux bundle a sacred ceremonial pipe in sage.

2. Bundle your sacred possessions—like a healing crystal, mineral, lodestone, or other stone—inside a sage bundle between uses.

3. Take a bath containing three to four drops clary sage, rosemary, eucalyptus, or pine. This is an ideal way of ridding the body of negative spirits that may have been encountered or accumulated on the person during smudging. I swear by this type of bath, and this is the way of practitioners of Santeria, Candomble, Vodou, Obeah, Hoodoo, and many other practices inspired by ATRs.

4. Essential oils can also work as a cleansing substitute for smudging. Add ½ teaspoon pine, juniper, fir, cedar, or spruce to a wash bucket filled with water. Add ¼ cup unscented Castile soap. Mix. Wash counter tops, bathrooms, floors, or walls to enjoy the herbal blessings of sacred evergreens during spring cleaning rites.

In closing, remember the African notion of *Iwa-pele*—always consider balance in any health ritual. That means that just as you smudge to banish negativity, you will want to add charms, natural amulets, and different types of drawing incenses to invite positive spirits by using affirmative herbs like life everlasting, frankincense, and myrrh.

CHAPTER TEN

Intergenerational Afro Care

Curly hair is beautiful, but it is also very complex. Sometimes we treat it forcefully, especially in an attempt to detangle—ultimately this is the wrong approach. Curly hair has a complicated hair shaft. Pull out a strand and examine it. I'm sure you will find variation in the width of the strand—at certain points it is quite thick, while in other areas it is thin. The irregularity in the hair shaft, especially at the thin points, makes it more likely to break if stressed than straight hair. Curly hair requires TLC.

Herbs and Curly Hair, a Caveat

In addition to saponin-rich natural shampoo herbs, other herbs can be added for various effects. One thing to remember, though, is that most herbs are astringent (drying). Many herbs popularly used for hair care are well suited to straight, oily hair but may challenge curly or kinky hair. This includes popular hair herbs like rosemary, sage, horsetail, and nettles. Secondly, although herbs are natural, they can still be irritating, drying, and can even cause a rash. Add herbs judiciously, one at a time, testing for allergic reactions. If your hair is described as coarse, kinky, nappy, or very thick, pay special attention to these warnings. Typically these types of hair tend to be dry. You may benefit from the addition of a teaspoon or two of olive oil, hempseed oil, neem, jojoba (a wax), or melted shea or mango butter when adding extra herbs. Herbs that release plant mucilage, burdock root, marshmallow root, slippery elm, and emollient comfrey retain moisture. If you suffer from frizziness and want to define your curls, add one teaspoon vegetable glycerin or aloe to the recipes.

Herbs used historically in natural shampoos include rosemary, sage, and walnut hulls for brunette or black hair; chamomile, calendula, and mullein for blond or light brown hair; rose hips, henna, hibiscus flowers, and cinnamon for red, auburn, or burgundy hair. Nettles, horsetail, and sea kelp nourish hair and strengthen it, thereby encouraging hair growth. Chamomile, comfrey, and catmint (catnip) soothe scalp irritation. Tea tree, garlic, onion, and neem are used as antibacterial, antifungal agents to deter scalp disorders and infections. Hops (one of the main herbs in beer; this is why beer rinses have been used for hundreds of years) and chamomile add body and thickness.

Saponins

Shampoo was not always formulated by chemists or in the factory; this is a very new approach that came into vogue during the late nineteenth and early twentieth centuries. Saponins are nature's sudsing agents and they are found in herbs. Saponin-rich herbs come from specific fruit trees, roots, flowers, and mineral-packed weeds.

Make Your Own Botanical Shampoo

Most herbs do not produce frothy lather, but who needs it anyway? The idea, particularly with curly hair, is to cleanse gently without stripping hair of sebum (natural oils). Listed below are some of nature's better cleansers.

Lamb's Quarter (*Chenopodium album*): A common North American and European weed, probably already lurking about in your garden, ready for harvest, lends mild cleansing action.

Papaya Leaf (*Carica papaya*): From the pawpaw tree, papaya leaf releases gentle cleansers when infused in hot water.

Soap bark tree (*Quillaja saponaria*): The bark, as it sounds, contains enough saponin to provide a good soap, useful as a shampoo. Barks need to be decocted, rather than infused.

Soapwort (*Saponaria officinalis*): is a weed that has been used for cleansing hair, the body, and fine textiles for centuries. Some museum preparators still use soapwort to cleanse ancient textiles. This attests to soapwort's mild, nurturing nature. To make soapwort shampoo or lingerie wash, infuse one cup soapwort in two cups water, covered for twenty minutes.

Yucca (*Yucca glauca, Y. baccata, Y. angustifolia*): Also called "soap root" and amole. Used in traditional rituals and rite-of-passage ceremonies in Mexico by the Hopi and a few other Southwest Indian communities, yucca is also used to deter dandruff, baldness, and thinning hair. Yucca needs to be pulverized and soaked before using.

Yucca, and sometimes its relatives from the *Agave* genus, such as *Agave lechuguilla*, are used to make shampoo, soap, and clothing detergent. To prepare for use, peel a young root so that only the white inside remains. Pound this using a large mortar and pestle, or use a mallet or hammer. Put bruised root inside a piece of muslin. Tie shut with rubber band or a piece of natural cotton string. Place in hot water. Work the root between your hands until the soapy substance is released into the water.

Why Bother?
Of course you and I know that it is easy to run out to the local shops and choose from a wide array of shampoos, so why bother?

Connection
Many people enjoy direct engagement with herbs, feeling that they benefit spirituality from contact with nature.

Avoiding Chemicals
Other people do not trust the plethora of chemicals used in shampoo formulas—these do-it-yourself types prefer to make their own from scratch.

Ecology and Sustainability

Some people want to participate in the natural ecology around them in a positive way. They would never use weed killer, for example, to kill lamb's quarter. Instead, they use the prolific weed for its nutrients in hair care formulas and in other holistic ways. Abundant leaves from the papaya tree can be used to make cleansers rather than simply disposed of when they fall from the tree. Making shampoo offers opportunities to reuse and recycle old squeeze-top bottles rather than discarding them. Homemade herbal brews bring satisfaction from growing, harvesting, and then using your own organic ingredients.

Ancient Traditions

Mexicans and Southwest Indians, notably the Hopi, have used yucca as an important element in beauty and rite-of-passage rituals, and in ceremonies during prenuptial rites. Many contemporary people feel that they too can benefit from these ancient traditions. Yucca is ideal for the rich brown and black, wavy, thick hair prevalent in Middle Eastern, African, southern European, Native American, and Latino ethnic groups. Soapwort and soapbark, along with lamb's quarter and papaya leaf, are gentle and effective cleansers, well suited to the delicate curly, kinky, or nappy hair.

Essential Oils for Healthy Hair

Essential oils are condensed organic ingredients that accentuate the effects of prepared shampoos. Aromatic botanical oils are regaining the popularity they enjoyed in early civilizations. They are well respected for their ability to address a variety of issues such as dull, dry, and thinning hair, as well as itchy, irritated scalp—these are aromatherapeutic benefits. The scents of essential oils provide a therapy of their own, sometimes referred to as aromacology because they affect our psychological makeup and mood. Since essential oils are highly concentrated, only a few drops are necessary to achieve great results. The following table is inspired by *The Complete Book of Essential Oils and Aromatherapy*, by esteemed aromatherapist Dr. Valerie Ann Worwood.[1] The table illustrates the suitability of essential oils for various types of hair.

Essential Oil for Hair

Essential Oils	Normal Hair	Dry Hair	Oily Hair	Fragile Hair
Birch (*Betula lenta*)		x	x	
Carrot (*Daucus carota*)	x		x	
Clary Sage (*Salvia sclarea*)				x
Eucalyptus Lemon (*Eucalyptus citriodora*)	x		x	
Lavender (*Lavandula angustifolium; L. officinalis*)	x	x	x	
Neroli (*Citrus bigaradia; C. aurantium*)	x			
Parsley (*Petroselinum sativum*)	x	x		x
Patchouli (*Pogostemon patchouli*)	x			
Peppermint (*Mentha piperita*)	x			
Rosemary (*Rosmarinus officinalis*)	x	x	x	
Sandalwood (*Santalum album*)		x		x
Tea Tree (*Melaleuca alternifolia*)	x		x	x
Yarrow (*Achillea millefolium*)		x	x	

Hydrosols

Hydrosols are the essences of fragrant plants extracted and preserved in distilled water. Aromatherapist of the Aromatic Plant Project, Jeanne Rose, coined the term hydrosol, though they are also referred to as floral waters. The three most popular hydrosols are:

> Rose (formerly called rose water): astringent, energizing, calming, fragrant

> Neroli (also called orange flower water): uplifting, hydrating, mellow

> Lavender (sometimes called lavender water): moisturizing, balancing, unisex

Hydrosols are the lightest natural hair sprays/moisturizers available. They work like a charm with Afros and other curly dos, especially when the emphasis is on enhancing natural curl, not controlling it. You can use them to replace some or all of the plain water used to create herbal shampoo, as in this recipe:

Relaxing Rhassoul Shampoo

¼ cup Moroccan rhassoul mud

½ cup rose water

½ cup orange flower water

7 drops neroli essential oil

5 drops sandalwood essential oil

3 drops patchouli essential oil

Put rhassoul mud in nonreactive bowl (Pyrex or stainless steel). Slowly whisk in hydrosols. Drop in essential oils. Whisk until smooth. Cover hair. Massage gently. Cover with plastic cap. Leave on fifteen to thirty minutes. Rinse well.

Shortcuts

Doctoring

With our busy lives, many people simply do not have the time to make personal care products themselves. If you fit into this group, yet want to add your own unique touches, "doctoring" is the right method for you. Doctoring is old slang for taking something that already exists and adding your own personal touches—suggestions follow:

Castile Soap

Castile soap is highly touted in homemade shampoo recipes. Castile soap is made from shredded olive oil soap, dissolved in water. It is widely available from health food stores and natural product suppliers.

Avgo Lemono Shampoo

Combine eight ounces Castile soap, two tablespoons strained lemon juice, and an egg yolk at room temperature. Blend all ingredients with whisk in a bowl. Add ⅛ teaspoon each lemon verbena and lemon essential oil. Whisk. Use immediately.

Shampoo Base

A popular option for those pressed for time is to purchase prepared shampoo bases that are unscented, natural, or organic and then add essential oils.

Tip: Add eight to sixteen drops (total) essential oils (refer to chart) to two cups shampoo base. If shampoo base is unavailable, try unscented baby shampoo.

Nutrients

You can also add ¼ cup dried, ground sea kelp or seaweed to emulsify (thicken) shampoo and add nourishment.

Dairy products, buttermilk, full-fat "real" mayonnaise, sour cream, or whole cream are softening natural ingredients that hydrate and help detangle. Pick one and add ¼ cup to strained, scented shampoo brew. Refrigerate the unused portion. Use within a week. Eggs are useful because they add body, shine, and protein. Always use at room temperature. Separate egg and just use the yolk for hair (it's easier to rinse out).

The great part about making your own hair care products is that you can experiment with the ingredients, adjusting them until they are perfectly suited to your hair texture. By tailoring the essential oils, you can create an alluring scent that is unique. Creating shampoo in bulk is economical, wholesome, and relaxing.

Locs: A Journey of Personal Transformation

Not long ago, the main places where you would see locs (sometimes called dreadlocks) were in Africa or the Caribbean, particularly Jamaica. For the Rastafarians of Jamaica, the Shaivas (devotees of Shiva) and Vaishnavas (devotees of Vishnu) of India, and numerous clans in Africa including the Turkana, the Massai, the Samburu of Kenya, the Himba of Namibia, the Fulani of Senegal, and the Baye Fall (Black Muslims), locked hair is not a hairstyle, it is a reflection of a way of life, grounded by culture, tradition, and most of all spirituality. Just as many different cultures have hair-locking traditions, so too does this distinctive way of wearing the hair have diverse names including *Natty Dreads* (Rastafarians), *Ndiagne* (Baye Falls), and *Jatta* (gurus of India).

Many people of Jamaican and African heritage have migrated and now live on the East Coast in and around New York City. It is in New

York that locked hair took a hold on popular culture, transcending its traditional connection to spirituality and faith to become a cultural statement with all people. Acclaimed author Alice Walker has worn locs for many years, and so have other artists including Bob Marley and Whoopi Goldberg.

In the beautifully illustrated book *Dreads*, Francesco Mastalia and Alfonse Pagano interviewed people from around the world about why their hair is worn in what they call "dreadlocks."[2] (Today, most people reject the combination of terms "dread" "lock" because it has negative connotations, particularly because of the word dread, which evokes fear.) As might be expected, there was a wide range of reasons, from strong faith-based cultural tradition to easy grooming, attraction to the style, and everything in between.

Decisions, Decisions

There are various schools of thought within the curly-topped community. Some folk long for straight hair and lean toward the tools, chemicals, and techniques that will give the desired effect. Others absolutely adore their curly locs and wouldn't have their hair any other way. These folks seek out products and techniques that will accentuate their curls or leave their hair to do what it will. Still others like their naturally curly hair but wish for an easier grooming regimen. For those individuals looking for relatively easy grooming and a natural look that is a throwback to Africa, or seeking connection to earth-based spiritual wisdom from around the world, locs are an ideal choice.

Many people, including myself, enjoy naturally curly hair but find a variety of challenges with maintenance of curly locs. Issues include the expense of products that promise to manage, enhance, or accentuate curly hair but often fall short. Curly hair, particularly of the densely coiled nature of African-descended people, is very resistant to change. While there are many excellent products on the market, African curls tend to have a mind of their own. Our curls naturally coil around each other, producing tangles. We don't have a hold on this phenomenon because people of various ethnicities have tightly curled or even wiry hair.

Many of us spend hours and indeed years, as well as thousands of dollars, to manage or prevent tangles. If we keep our hair short, it is lovely and generally manageable. This is an ideal situation for tightly curled hair. The tangles of shorter hair are easier to manage, but they can become quite a bit more challenging with longer hair. The battle of the tangles, or as we typically call them, naps, leads to breakage. Long nappy hair that is tightly curled often becomes uneven, damaged, and ultimately frustrating. For individuals with tightly curled hair that tends to tangle, snarl, or nap up, locs are an ideal choice, particularly if you also desire longer hair.

Grooming with Spirit, Purpose, and Patience

Patience is an issue that arises, even for those with ideal hair for locs, which would be hair that is tightly curled without any chemical straighteners. For these individuals, locs can take at least six months to become permanent. For those with looser curls or wavy hair, it could take two years. If you can be mindful and focus on the end result, this time will be a part of a larger metamorphosis within that allows change to occur at its own rate. Some people will find yoga and meditation especially helpful as well because it encourages a focus within rather than on outward appearance.

Social and Psychological Implications

The appearance of locked hair evokes a wide variety of responses. Some people find locs suggestive of the counterculture or to be radically different from their personal orientation. If these people exert control over your life, whether they are your parents, administrators, advisors, or a boss at work, you will need to enter into a meaningful conversation during your transformation. Sometimes there are so many issues that go much deeper than hair that a conversation may have been long overdue. Talking can help strengthen and develop stronger ties. You will need to weigh your priorities and if it turns out that your priority is the locked hair and those around you strongly reject the idea, you will need to evaluate how to proceed.

The Nitty-Gritty

Once you decide to lock your hair, you will of course need more than anything to be patient. I started my locs—or rather, they started themselves—approximately a year ago. They are still not all the way locked because my curls are loose. I twist them regularly but not fanatically, and I see a loctian when possible. A good loctian is indispensable, especially early on in the process when the locs are being established. She will clean your scalp well, condition your hair, re-part your hair, and carefully twist or roll the hair. Having a skilled loctian is a great way of keeping a very neat look.

One of the most highly recommended technical books for those trying to establish locs is *Plaited Glory: For Colored Girls Who've Considered Braids, Locks, and Twists* by Lonnice Brittenum Bonner.[3] Another popular book, *No More Lye: The African American Woman's Guide to Natural Haircare* by Tulani Kinard, gives practical advice for beginning locs naturally. Kinard advises readers to part the hair evenly in small pieces of about a half-inch, and to either palm roll, twist, or braid each segment tightly.[4] These twists or braids should be left alone for at least one month. After this time period, the hair can be washed, with an emphasis on cleansing the scalp rather than the hair itself. Some people cleanse their scalp with natural herbs like a witch hazel tincture in between shampoos to feel fresher. After about one month the hair is shampooed, re-rolled or twisted, held down with hair clips, and dried under a hair dryer or naturally in sunlight. This is repeated for many months until the hair is permanently locked. According to Kinard, the ideal method is for a hollow core to form at the center of each loc and for the hair to be encouraged to curl around this core. This allows light and airy locs, which move freely and have a natural sheen that are also easy to clean. The problem with the quick and easy methods, particularly those promoted for use on straighter hair, is that the hair gets irreparably dirty and by using grease or wax the locs actually become dirt magnets. Moreover there is not a natural, light, and airy hollow core to the hair; it is simply clumped together and can be quite unattractive.

I am a do-it-yourself type. I had been wearing two-stranded twists for about three years, and when they started to lock up I embraced the possibility of physical transformation. Eventually, I did seek out the expertise of several loctians and I was grateful to have some of the messy areas sorted out. You can find a loctian in most major cities, and typically they advertise as "Natural Haircare Salons." There are numerous products available to help manage your locs, though it is a personal choice, just like the decision whether or not to consult a loctian. Generally, less is more with locs. My loctian, who is an Igbo person from Nigeria, even warns against naturally oily ingredients like shea butter or lanolin for loc maintenance because they weigh down the locs and attract dirt.

The essential tools for locs are as follows:

1. A rat-tailed comb to part and roll the hair.

2. A light, clear shampoo such as Johnson and Johnson's Baby Shampoo or a salon brand containing essential oils like lavender or chamomile.

3. A natural conditioner, either homemade or from a manufacturer that promotes natural essential oils, for example Aveda or African Root Stimulator.

4. A water-based gel that obviously does not contain heavy waxes or oils. Try Natural Root Stimulator Lock and Twisting Gel or create your own, simply using pure aloe vera and water, applied in dime-sized portions.

5. Patience, patience, patience.

Remember that even with locs, it's not the destination but the journey itself that can lead to personal transformation.

Mother and Daughter Natty Hair Rituals

Since the beginning of time, people have enjoyed the benefits of rituals. Africans in particular have combined herbs and rituals such as relaxing head massage. Today, Indian head massage (*Malish*) is enjoying attention in the United States.

I grew up as a "tender-headed" child. I, like many people with thick, tightly curled, easily tangled long hair, readily feel pain and am not shy about letting everyone know about it. The word "ouch," followed by a flood of tears, was synonymous with hair washing time and with being tender-headed during my youth.

Today, as an herbalist and aromatherapist, I have discovered numerous ways of easing pain naturally. Mother and daughter benefit from bonding, trust, affection, and sharing. The simple rituals shared in this chapter, paired with herbal remedies, encourage gentle hair care. Ingredients listed are useful for African-descended children with tightly curled, kinky, or nappy hair.

Soothing Ritual

1. Put on a melodic CD—try Bobby McFerrin, Sweet Honey in the Rock, or Ladysmith Black Mambazo on African Lullaby by Music for Little People.

2. Warm sweet almond, jojoba, avocado oil, or shea butter in a microwave or on a stovetop.

3. Have the child sit on a zafu or zabuton (Zen meditation pillows). These types work especially well, though any pillow will do.

4. Retrieve oil from microwave or stovetop. Add three drops lavender, sandalwood, or chamomile essential oil or one drop rose otto to accentuate the relaxing nature of the oil. Situate yourself so that your child is between your knees on her pillow. Dip your fingers into the oil and gently massage her entire scalp.

5. Put a plastic cap on her head or wrap her hair in cellophane. Wrap again in large towel. Have the child lie down on the pillow and listen to relaxing music for twenty minutes.

6. Light nag champa or another pleasing incense; place in censer or fireproof holder.

7. Shampoo hair using a high-quality detangling shampoo, such as Cream of Nature. Towel dry.

8. Put a clean dry towel around her neck. Mist hair with No More Tangles.

9. Mist her face and hair again, this time using lavender or rose water. Mist your face as well; repeat when you encounter snarls.

10. Separate wet hair with an Afro pick; mist as needed. Style, using the widest comb available.

Gentle Styling Ideas

The blessing of kinky and curly hair is the numerous styling options. Moms or other caretakers can allow individuality and creativity to shine. Each style becomes a makeover and an adventure. Here are a few options that are easy for you, gentle to children's scalp, and well suited to African hair.

1. Use a soft headband or colorful scarf folded down to headband size. Put the hair into a softly sculpted puff by shaping it with your hands.

2. Part the hair in the middle and make two Afro puffs if the hair is long enough. Use a scrunchie. For added fun, make a zigzag part.

3. For a longer lasting hairstyle, try a double strand twist:

   › Looking down at the top of the head, divide the hair into four sections.

   › Clip or braid three of the four sections individually to contain the hair.

   › Part the hair into ¾-inch squares; twist (using two strands).

- › Apply aloe vera gel to the hair to hold ends and keep them from unravelling, or if necessary use matching rubber bands.

- › Take breaks. Massage her shoulders. Mist hair and apply aloe as needed. Continue until the entire head is styled. This hairstyle should last at least four weeks, especially if a silk scarf is worn to bed or if silk or satin pillowcases are used.

Fait Accompli

Complete the ritual with a cup of peppermint or chamomile tea:

Boil two cups water; add one Celestial Seasons peppermint or chamomile tea bag to each cup; pour water over tea bags, filling cup. Sweeten with honey and flavor with lemon or milk if desired.

By now, the two of you should be relaxed and eagerly looking forward to next month's ritual. In the interim, have fun shopping for interesting oils, incense, herbs, and floral waters for the next mother and daughter hair ritual.

Herbal Dyes for Mature African Hair

As we grow older, our hair gradually turns gray, losing its natural color. For some, this process begins as early as the twenties. Many women are not ready for such a big change. Some want to hold onto their natural hair color, while others choose to enhance gray or white hair. Like most dark fibers, brunette or black hair is more resistant to dyes than light fibers or blonde hair. The complex hair shaft of kinky and curly hair requires more colorant, and gray hair is very resistant. To top it off, hair grows a quarter to a half inch per month, making coloring hair a challenge.

Shown resistance, we have a tendency to reach for permanent color rather than gentle solutions—this can lead to damage, especially if relaxers or straighteners are also used. This section is written for those seeking natural ways to enrich graying hair. Botanical rinses work with existing color, providing subtle highlights, increased shine, and youthful vibrancy without permanent changes.

Red Hot Oil

Reddish highlights warm sallow skin and enliven dingy gray hair. A rich red hue can be created from the roots of the herb alkanet (*Alkanna tinctoria*), extracted into oil. Red Hot Oil conditions dry hair and colors it simultaneously. Apply as a hot oil treatment.

⅓ cup alkanet root, cut and sifted
⅔ cup sweet almond, safflower, or olive oil

Yield: two or more applications (depending on hair length)

Place the alkanet root in a sterile, dry jar with screw top. Fill jar with oil. Set in window. Steep twenty-four hours; swirl periodically. Warm ¼ cup red oil. Divide hair into four sections. Part hair ¼ inch at a time and apply heated oil from roots to tip. Put on plastic cap; then wrap head in towel. Leave on forty-five minutes, then shampoo. Red Hot Oil has a shelf life of one year.

Flamin' Red

This recipe features madder root (*Rubia tinctorum*) a relative of alkanet root featured in the previous recipe. Flamin' Red works well on medium or dark brown hair. As progressive dye, color intensifies with repeated use.

1½ cups water
⅓ cup madder root
2 tablespoons apple cider vinegar

Makes: approximately twelve ounces.

Boil water. Add madder root. Stir; cover; reduce heat to medium. Simmer thirty minutes. Add vinegar, then simmer thirty more minutes. Reduce heat to low; steep one hour more. Strain. Cool. See catch method on page 116 for application procedure. Flamin' Red has a very short shelf life; use within twenty-four hours.

Henna

One of the strongest hair dyes is henna (*Lawsonia inermis*). People have enjoyed henna since the civilizations of ancient Egypt. As legend has it, Cleopatra had lovely red hair, as did Nefertiti. Henna brings out reddish highlights in the most resistant hair, including graying hair. Henna is not recommended for hair that has been dyed recently with commercial dyes because a chemical reaction can occur, turning hair black. Henna is also not recommended for hair more than fifty percent gray. To use packaged types, follow manufacturer's directions and enhance as follows:

Henna Hints

> Shampoo hair first.

> Enhance red tones by using cognac, red wine, carrot juice, cranberry juice, hibiscus tea, or rosehip tea in place of water.

> Tint and scent: add vanilla extract for scent or any combination of ground allspice, cinnamon, or cloves for enriched brown tones. Limit spices to a teaspoon. Avoid use on abraded or sensitive scalps, or if you are allergic to these ingredients.

> Minimize brassiness—use strong black coffee, rosemary, sage, or black tea in place of the water.

> For body, add flat beer or hops tea in place of water.

> Quench dryness with the addition of mayonnaise.

> Attract moisture with yogurt, sour cream, honey, or molasses.

> Follow up with a hot oil treatment to counteract dryness.

Rosemary (*Rosmarinus officinalis*) and Sage (*Salvia officinalis*) Rinse

This is an age-old formula for blending gray hair into darkly colored hair. It works on the same principle as tea or coffee—staining, facilitated by the concentration of tannins.

½ cup distilled water
1 teaspoon dried rosemary
1 teaspoon dried sage

Boil water; add the herbs. Cover; reduce the heat to medium. Simmer twenty minutes. Reduce heat to low; simmer twenty minutes. Turn off heat; steep one hour. Strain. Apply using the catch method (see page 116). This recipe yields approximately twelve ounces has a shelf life of two weeks.

Alternative: use three cups strong coffee or black tea. To prepare: brew three tablespoons loose Assam, Ceylon, or oolong tea or three Tetley tea bags in three cups boiled water. Cool. Apply using the catch method.

Tobacco Herbal Rinse

Tobacco (*Nicotiana* spp.) rinse is one of the most effective ways of quickly staining graying hair. This rinse adds golden, auburn tones.

1½ cup distilled water
¼ cup dried tobacco
2 tablespoons vinegar

Boil water; add tobacco. Reduce heat to medium-low; cover. Infuse forty minutes. Remove from heat; add vinegar; steep twenty minutes. Strain. Apply using the catch method. This recipe yields approximately twelve ounces and has a shelf life of one month, refrigerated.

Nights on Negril Beach

This is natural bluing designed to bring a midnight moonlit glow to graying hair. This will also enrich black hair.

2 cups water
½ cup blueberries
½ cup blackberries
pinch salt
2 tablespoons powdered alum

Boil water. Add berries, salt, and alum. Cover; reduce heat to medium. Simmer twenty minutes, checking, stirring, and mashing berries every few minutes. Strain through a fine sieve. Apply using the catch method.

Hot Shea Butter Hair Treatment

Shea is a good hot oil treatment, wherein it is melted, cooled slightly, then applied warm to the ends of hair (where split ends occur) and to the scalp. Use a clean art paintbrush as a handy tool for applying the warmed oil to scalp. Part hair in sections as you work. Work quickly, otherwise shea will solidify. Put on a plastic cap, and sit out in the sun if possible or under a dryer for thirty minutes. Alternatively, cover your head with a bath towel to retain heat. After a half-hour, shampoo thoroughly and rinse. Shea adds shine and softens.

Hair Pomade

Africans have been using shea butter as a hair dressing for hundreds of years. This application is recommended for super thick, curly, kinky, or dry hair. Thin, straight hair would become overwhelmed and weighed down by a shea pomade; locs may also appear dull or develop a tendency to attract dirt when shea is applied, so it is not recommended for them.

Scoop out about a teaspoon of shea butter in the palm of your hands (use less for short hair and more for longer hair). Place your palms together. Rub gently, using your body heat to melt the shea butter. Once shea transforms from solid to liquid, rub on your hair, then style as usual. This is fine as a weekly hair dressing pomade.

Botanical Styling Gel

A very effective gel can be created from flaxseed or Irish moss since both contain mucilage. I have used both many times with great success. They add body and shine without the flakiness of some commercial products. They also cost a fraction of the price of prepared products from beauty salons or drugstores.

1 teaspoon Irish moss or ground flaxseed
¾ cup water
¼ cup vodka
1 teaspoon essential oil, absolute, or hydrosol

Dissolve one teaspoon cut and sifted Irish moss or ground flaxseed in ¾ cup water. You will need to adjust the amount by doubling or tripling the quantity if you have long or very thick hair. Put in a pot. Bring to a boil. Stir. Add more botanical or water ratio given, if needed. Stir. Reduce heat to medium and continue to cook for eight minutes. Remove from heat. Whisk in vodka and scent of your choice. I suggest neroli, rose, lavender, patchouli, or a mixture. Whisk again. Leave to set up overnight. You can apply this to freshly washed hair and it will help define curls and hold hair into smooth up-dos or chignons, or you can use it as a setting lotion as you would a commercial lotion.

Now that we have partaken in spring activities for the mind, body, and spirit, it is time to move on to summer's cornucopia of goodness.

Summer

CHAPTER ELEVEN

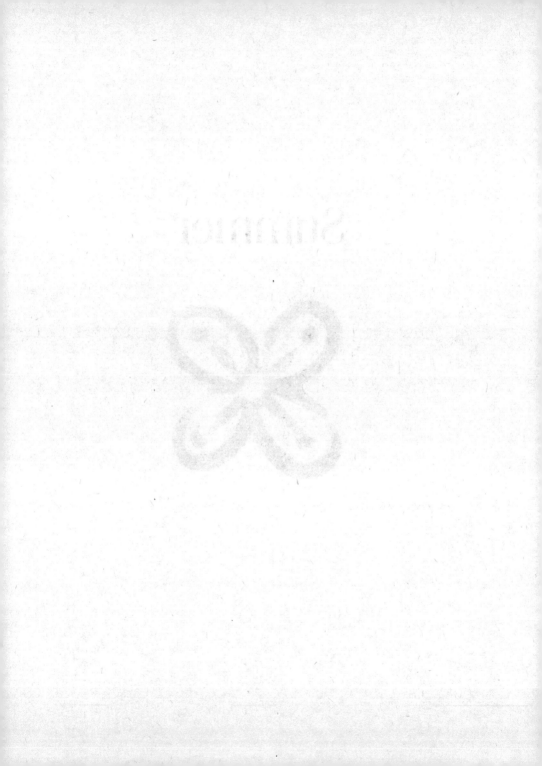

Blossoms of Love, Youth, and Vibrant Health

Summer: Magic with Herbs and the Orisha

Summer is a flurry of activity. It is a season that is particularly important to our holistic health. Summer is the time we can build our reserve of mojo for the rest of the year. It is a time of planting seeds, early harvests of herbs, and general abundance. Summer is also the time when we come out of our shells, meeting with old friends and new folks. It affords us time to step out of ourselves, recognizing what we have in common, reaching across boundaries, and extending community through an appreciation of nature.

The beauty of trees speaks to us on a very deep level, awakening our senses of sight, smell, and sound through their flowers, new leaves, and movement. We should take this cue to awaken our collective spiritual energy, realizing the ways trees are celebrated across diverse cultures. This in turn allows us to see our common appreciation of their sacred nature, giving us an additional way to connect culturally.

The Yoruba people make groves, which are regarded as sacred. These groves honor deities and serve as consecrated workshops called "Igboro groves," sacred to the spirit of the ancestors. Another type of

grove is one specifically for the orisha, for example the Igbo Osayin—
the sacred grove of Osayin. Taboos, based on spirituality and traditional value systems, have protected the trees of various communities
in Africa, including the Malshegu community of the northern region
of Ghana.

Magic of Oak

The oak tree is associated with the Druids who are thought to have con-
gregated in oak groves. Northwestern Europeans also found the oak to
be of symbolic importance. Oak, called *Duir* in Celtic, is often associated with summer solstice. It represents strength, endurance, and forti-
tude. The oak tree is the door between the light and dark halves of the
year; the oak door connects us with the other world. It is sacred to the
Druids because of its tendency to attract lightning and survive lightning strikes by regenerating readily afterward.

Oak Moon is based on what is known of the old Celtic Tree Month
observations, which have now been connected with full moons. The
time when Oak Moon occurs varies each year and can range from mid-
June to early July. One of the treasures, evident during Oak Moon, is
that the leaves of the tree are a bright, almost crayon green, and are
shaped like outstretched human hands. The leaves feel tender to the
touch and they smell fresh. Oak Moon affords an opportunity to engage
in dynamic strength, the wonder of nature, the spirit of renewal, and the
commitment to deities or a spiritual path. As we delve into summer, we
do so going through the magical oak door.

This hardy tree is steeped in mysticism and holds the spirit of the
ancestors, as it is a tree linked to ancient rites and celebrations of many
groups of people on both sides of the Atlantic from various lineages.
Across cultures, oak is revered for its longevity and strength, and is considered a reservoir of perennial knowledge. The sacred oak tree represents the Great Mother; it is our link to other worlds and to different
groups of people.

Oak Moon Bathing Ritual

To absorb some of the nurturing gifts of oak, go outside and gather ten pliable oak leaves. Draw a bath at dusk. Light a white candle with the scent of rain; place this on a safe candleholder. Place seven of the leaves in the tub. Use the other three to wash your body. Wet, then lather up one leaf at a time and wash your body as you recite:

Strength and courage I summon thee

Wisdom of the mighty oak tree

Cleanse me, treat me, and touch my soul

Thereby others I can make whole

Juneteenth: Working for Freedom

A few weeks after Oak Moon, a little-known holiday commemorating a curious event in American history arrives. June nineteenth, which is called Juneteenth, marks the delayed transmittal of the news of emancipation to enslaved Africans held in Texas. Whatever your ethnicity, it is always good to recognize that you have freedom—or if not, Juneteenth reminds you to work hard at obtaining it.

If there are bonds tying you down, such as debt, addictions, or unwanted relationships, create a list that marks out a strategy that leads toward freedom. Wear white on Juneteenth—it is the color of spiritual strength. Fire is important. For dinner, have a barbeque featuring your favorite foods. Be sure to include some tasty roasted tubers and root veggies like sweet potato and sweet onion. Have an extravagant soft drink—it is the tradition to have strawberry soda, but some of you working hard to improve your health will want to reach for berry-flavored mineral water, sparkling cranberry juice, or a strawberry-banana smoothie instead. As the coals of the fire turn white with heat and the sun settles in the west it is time to turn to ritual. It is appropriate to purge things holding you down. Burn old unnecessary papers. Set yourself free from the past by clearing clutter. You'd be surprised how much this improves your mental health!

Freedom from Addiction and the Chains that Bind Mojo

The Fourth of July is the date when the Declaration of Independence was officially adopted by Congress in 1776. One of the more compelling portions of the declaration, particularly in relation to women and people of color is *We hold these truths to be self-evident, that all men are created equal, that they are endowed by their Creator with certain unalienable Rights, that among these are Life, Liberty and the pursuit of Happiness.* Clearly though, this beautiful sentiment did not apply to all of us as it was not until 1863 that the Emancipation Proclamation was written, stating *That on the first day of January, in the year of our Lord one thousand eight hundred and sixty-three, all persons held as slaves within any State or designated part of a State, the people whereof shall then be in rebellion against the United States, shall be then, thenceforward, and forever free; and the Executive Government of the United States, including the military and naval authority thereof, will recognize and maintain the freedom of such persons, and will do no act or acts to repress such persons, or any of them, in any efforts they may make for their actual freedom.* Later still, the Nineteenth Amendment of the Constitution was ratified, finally giving women the right to vote, *The right of citizens of the United States to vote shall not be denied or abridged by the United States or by any State on account of sex.*

All the while, there has been a humble root, dug up from the depths of our Great Mother that Hoodoos of various faiths, colors, and creeds have held close to their person. This root is typically shrouded inside a mojo bag. It is emblematic of freedom and personal rights, and it holds the promise of happiness. We call it High John the Conqueror (*Ipomoea jalapa*). It is more than a simple tuber; it is held tight in a *hand*, also called a mojo bag, as a symbolic representation of breaking free of the chains of slavery. High John, a relative of both morning glory and the sweet potato, represents the slave who could not be held in chains, who fights the endless war against enslavement until freedom is obtained.

We all suffer from one type of slavery or another. Today, create a mojo, utilizing the power of the natural amulet, High John, along with the stone hematite, known to strengthen the system and help one break free of addictions. Nestle various supplemental natural ingredients into the bag, and you have a potent mojo on your hands.

Get yourself a red flannel bag with a drawstring closure and add in a High John the Conqueror root. Add a clear, charged, powerful-feeling hematite stone. Put a pinch of kosher salt into the bag and a few devil's shoestrings to keep evil at bay. "Devil's shoestrings" actually refers to a number of species of viburnum: *Viburnum alnifolium* (alder-leafed viburnum or hobblebrush), *Viburnum opulus* (cramp-bark), or *Viburnum prunifolium* (black haw). These plants are in the honeysuckle family and all of them grow in the woods. Slippery elm, lemongrass, and eucalyptus are also known to aid in freedom, so throw in a little pinch of each. Roll the bag on the ground a few times so the herbs crumble and are well mixed. Finally, add a few drops of rose oil to feed the herbs, stones, and minerals (this will help them to stay powerful). Now you've got yourself a Freedom from Addiction and the Chains that Bind mojo bag. With this seasonal mojo close to your person, walk on, mindful of the treasure that we call freedom.

Mid-Summer Attraction Work

As you approach mid-summer you are bound to become a little more frisky, romantically inclined, or at the very least outgoing. Some people know just what to do to make their nature rise so that they are attractive to others. In case you need a few pointers, here are a few herbs sure to keep your mojo on track.

› Dab pure sandalwood oil on pulse points to attract people of the opposite sex. Sandalwood also calms nerves; it is relaxing and eases sexual inhibitions.

› Men, especially in the Middle East and North Africa, find Gulhina—the perfume oil of henna plant—a sure-fire way to become more attractive. It is used the same way as sandalwood oil.

- In Hoodoo and some other paths, folks who want to attract those of the same sex employ the assistance of lavender. I spoke about the balance of male/female energy found in lavender in my first book, Sticks, Stones, Roots & Bones. If you desire some same-sex loving, dab some lavender onto a few of your chakras, focus on your intent, go out and about, and see what happens.

- Southerners have taught us that the plants that grow so readily in their region can add a touch of magic to the love life. One such glorious herb comes from the fragrant magnolia tree. Slip a dried magnolia leaf or two between your mattress and box spring or under your futon to keep your lover close and faithful.

Little John, Justice Herb

One just can't help but reflect on our laws and the constitution during the summer months, because so many important amendments were enacted during these months. July 28 is the day the Fourteenth Amendment was enacted. The Fourteenth Amendment promises equal protection and due process of the law.

This is a great time to engage the herb beloved by Hoodoos. It is called Little John. Little John (*Alpina galanga*), also called galangal, is an herbal symbol of fairness and justice in legal proceedings. Unfortunately, sometimes equal protection and justice is not granted as promised, so we need extra help from the domain of the spirit. Here are a few ways Little John, a relative of ginger, can be used as a chew or charm in spell work:

- Put a cleaned piece of Little John into your mouth. Chew it until soft. Try not to swallow.

- If you are supporting a court case or are on trial, spit the Little John fluid outside the courthouse.

> If you want only good outcomes from legal proceedings by mail, spit the Little John juice near your post box.

> If you want a lawsuit you've been informed of by mail to end peacefully, spit on the envelope and bury it either at the crossroads or on your personal property.

> To positively influence the court, keep Little John on your person inside a red mojo bag, along with some calendula flowers, deer's tongue, and oregano.

Working Basil's Magical Green Energy

The fields and forest are bustling with every possible type of green by late July. Green is symbolic of verdant earth and abundance. Osayin's herbal delights and the fecundity of the Earth Mother reign supreme in July. Basil is an easy-to-grow summer green. It is always nice to find new ways to utilize it so it doesn't go to seed, because it grows prolifically. Try this floor wash with a fresh, crisp scent like green grass to harvest the abundance that is your destiny.

Add two cups fresh basil to a large cauldron of boiling water (use a stockpot if necessary). Remove the cauldron from heat. Add one ounce of pyrite chips to the cauldron. Cover. Set outside overnight. Strain; be careful to remove and save the pyrite for other spells. Add eight drops holy basil essential oil. Put a bowl of fine sea salt in the center of the room you are blessing. Cleanse surfaces with this Abundance Floor Wash using a natural sea sponge, with your dominant hand, concentrating on your desires the entire time. Sprinkle some of the fine sea salt on stains as you work. Open the doors and windows if possible so the spirits can aid your work. Good fortune should flow your way.

Ogun and Goofer Dust Protection Magic

With doors and windows ajar, and people coming and going with the breeze, one's attention might turn to natural protection magic in the summer. You can build your psychic armor utilizing the protective energy of orisha Ogun's warrior magic using goofer dust. Borrow this traditional formula from the Hoodoos. Add it to your repertoire of home and hearth protective potions. Take time out of your busy day to make and use some of this fierce protective dust.

Goofer dust is designed to protect your space from hants (disruptive spirits) and negative human energy. Mix equal parts sulfur (brimstone), sea salt, cayenne powder, and black pepper (powdered) and you'll have homemade goofer dust. Make enough of the powder for the job at hand. You'll want to spread this in a protective ring around your property. If it is an apartment, loft, or condo, make enough to spread out in front of your door. This dusts protects the home, blowing forcefully toward bad energy spread by intruders with malicious intentions.

Late Summer, Sun Ra Invocation

As the sun pierces your consciousness and you struggle through those dog days of summer, it becomes easy to understand the ancient Egyptian respect for the sun god, Ra. In the past, sunny days have helped you enjoy the fruits of summer and perhaps brought some romance and good health along the way. As I have said with the example of the rain, it's best to go with the spiritual mojo of each season. Shield your skin with an excellent sunscreen, but open your spiritual being fully to Ra.

Pay tribute to Ra for his blessings in the way he likes best. In ancient Egypt, myrrh was burned at high noon to please him. Put a few small chunks of myrrh on a white charcoal block placed on a fireproof surface outdoors. Use your hands to gently brush the smoke upward toward the heavens as you chant:

> In honor and praise I send this smoke toward you
>
> Thanks for the blessings and the sunny days, too
>
> Sun Ra, great god, emblem of the sun
>
> I honor and praise you for all that you've done

A Day of Peace

Summer has many themes. It is the season of freedom, justice, and peace. Within our war-torn world, September 19, the International Day of Peace, has all the more meaning. Try invoking the spirit of the Egyptian goddess Ma'at, whose primary purpose is to ensure fairness, justice, and peace.

Ma'at is actually one of my favorite goddesses. She weighs our hearts against an ostrich feather, creating a scale of justice. If equilibrium is struck between the feather and the heart, the person lived a good/just life and can pass on for a fruitful afterlife. If the heart is too heavy with remorse, the opposite occurs.

Use Ma'at's magical tool to bring clarity and peacefulness into your life. Touch all of your ceremonial tools with an ostrich feather today (if an ostrich feather is unavailable, it is fine to use a peacock feather as a substitute). Touch your correspondence, particularly legal papers, judgments, or liens with the feather of Ma'at so that people will deal with you in a just manner, ensuring peace and freedom. This completes projects for the spiritual atmosphere in the natural home. Now, we move on to the belly, as we explore ways of preparing seasonal soul food.

CHAPTER TWELVE

A Roast to Good Health

Roasting African-Caribbean Fruit and Vegetables

This is just a partial list of gifts of Africa and the diaspora. These foods are soulful and healthful; they also make wonderful additions to outdoor meals. Here is a short list along with preparation suggestions:

Banana: Place banana on grill with skin intact. Turn it until it is deep brown all the way around. Cut open to reveal baked banana. Serve with cold whipped cream and a touch of cinnamon for contrasting temperatures, color, and flavor.

Roasted Corn: Put corn with husk and silk intact on the grill away from flames. Turn periodically—about fifteen minutes. Shuck the corn and remove the silk. Eaten as is, roasted corn has a rustic smoky flavor. Tasty toppings range from the expected butter and sea salt to the more interesting serving suggestions I learned from my Latino friends. Squeeze the juice of a lemon or lime on the corn in place of salt. Try a dash of ground red pepper, a splash of hot sauce or a sprinkle of parmesan cheese to take it from a side dish to a main course. This is a vegetarian delight.

Grilled Pineapple: Peel pineapple; slice width-wise in half-inch slices. Place them directly on the grill. Sear each side about four minutes. Eat as an accompaniment to seafood or fish, or as a dessert.

COCONUT: THE FLESH FIT FOR OBATALA

Obatala, wise man, elder, orisha of all orishas, prefers the pure white flesh of coconut as an offering. Many may look at the stubborn brown hull and wonder how to get inside. Here are tips for selecting, opening, and creating basic milk from the coconut. This coconut milk has numerous purposes and can be used in the recipe for stuffed papaya roast.

Selection: Choose a coconut with a chestnut-brown hull that is smooth with no apparent holes or mold. Shake and listen for a water sound. If it still contains water, it will be moist and tasty.

Opening the Nut: Bore two holes in the eyes using an ice pick or sharp knife. The eyes are the dark brown spots at either end of the coconut. Pour coconut water into a bowl. You can add this to your bath or beauty recipes, or use it in rituals and ceremonies that honor appropriate orishas. Hit the hull on a hard surface sharply a few times—it should crack open.

You can also hit the nut with a mallet or hammer. Once cracked open, scoop out the flesh, which is called coconut meat, to use in the recipes that follow.

Making Coconut Milk: Heat 1½ cups water in a kettle on medium-high heat. Meanwhile, grate the coconut flesh and put it in a sieve over a large bowl. Just before the water comes to a boil, slowly pour it over the grated coconut in the sieve. Press the coconut meat with the back of a wooden spoon. Remove the sieve. Pour this liquid into a Pyrex measuring cup with a pouring spout. Repeat this step three to four times. This makes about 1¼ cups rich coconut milk.

Coconut Cream: To make coconut cream, bring 1½ cups full-fat milk almost to a boil. Go through steps above (making of coconut milk). Coconut cream is a bit denser, with a full-bodied, sweeter taste, just right for desserts and drinks.

Toasted Coconut: Remove coconut from the hull with a sharp knife. Shred the coconut. Add one tablespoon olive oil to a cast iron skillet. Add a pinch of sea salt if desired. Add the coconut and toss until medium brown. Toasted coconut is a great low-carb snack. I like to toast almonds and sunflower seeds with it and use this as a snack food when watching movies. You can also use toasted coconut as a topping for fruit salads, yogurt, or cereal.

Roasted Squash: You can roast summer squash, such as patty pan, chayote, zucchini, or hard-shelled winter squash like butternut, delicata, or acorn. Summer squash should be clean and dry. Then cook whole, slice, and add to kabobs, or chop and cook inside foil with olive oil, and season to taste. Summer squash can also be cut in half, the seeds and insides removed, brushed with corn, peanut, or olive oil, and seasoned with lemon, sea salt, and pepper. Ground ginger or cinnamon goes well with winter squash as well. Place prepared winter squash halves in foil. Put them on the barbeque grill. Roast until tender, about thirty-five to forty minutes.

Roasted Sweet Potato: Scrub the potato, rinse it, and pat it dry. Prick it with a fork. Wrap it in foil. Place it on grill. Turn periodically. It cooks in about half an hour on a medium grill. Test for doneness; it should feel soft. Cut it open. Carve an X shape on each half. Squeeze and fluff potato. Serve warm with butter, sea salt, fresh ground pepper, cinnamon, and cayenne. Roasted sweet potato with a dash of spice is sure to add nice warmth to a chilly eve.

Stuffed Papaya Roast

This is my adaptation of a hearty Caribbean dish, chock-full of antioxidants, vitamins, minerals, color, and a pungent curried flavor. Perfect for those who want to reduce meat intake but who are not yet ready to go all the way.

4-6 pound ripe Mexican papaya
½ teaspoon sesame oil
2 teaspoons corn oil, divided

2 cloves minced garlic

½ pound mushrooms

½ teaspoon sea salt

Freshly ground multicolored peppercorns

2 cups chicken broth

2 cups coconut milk

1 teaspoon cumin

1 teaspoon turmeric

½ teaspoon chili powder

2 cups white rice

½ cup mozzarella cheese, divided

½ cup parmesan cheese, divided

2 teaspoons butter chopped

Preheat oven to 350 degrees. Use a nonstick cooking sheet (if unavailable, spray a cooking sheet with vegetable oil spray or grease lightly with corn oil). Cut the papaya in half. Scoop out and discard seeds. Wash then pat papaya dry with towel; set it on the pan and set aside. Meanwhile, heat sesame oil and one teaspoon of the corn oil in a cast iron skillet on medium (vegetable spray is fine). Add garlic to the skillet. Wash mushrooms thoroughly. Chop coarsely. Add to the garlic; sauté the two ingredients. Add a pinch of sea salt and freshly ground pepper. Put mushroom/garlic blend, broth, coconut milk, spices, the remaining teaspoon of corn oil, and the rice into a rice cooker. Turn on "cook." If you don't have a cooker, add the ingredients (mushroom, garlic, broth, milk, spices, oil, rice) and follow the rice-cooking directions on page 61. When the rice is done, pour into a mixing bowl. Add half of the cheeses. Stir. Stuff the flavored rice into papaya shells. Top with remaining cheese and dot with the butter. Bake thirty to thirty-five minutes or until bubbly and top browns. Serve hot with salad.

I recommend the rainbow or multicolored peppercorns in soul food recipes because of their complex taste. They are actually berries grown in India and Borneo that mostly come from the same plant. The color variation is created by harvesting at different times during the growing season—green produces a fresh and pungent flavor, black has quite a bite, and white is more subtle. The pink is not a true peppercorn, yet it is added for its sweet, gentle heat.

This chapter was designed to help you develop creative ways of utilizing wholesome summer soul foods. Next, we move on to consider ways to engage summer to cultivate beauty.

CHAPTER THIRTEEN

Love, Sensuality, and Beauty

Iemanja is the mermaid orixa of the Afro-Brazilian path of Umbanda. She is the Brazilian manifestation of Yemaya-Ologun, whom I speak of so often as she is my patron orisha. Iemanja is so revered that she is seen as an incarnation of the Virgin Mary by a culture that is largely Catholic. She is the one to turn to when you are near the sea, since it is her home.

In warm weather, devotees petition Iemanja for good fortune by the seaside. Our minds frequently turn to her during the summer months when so much love and natural beauty surround us. People come bearing gifts for blessings during the coming year. In Hoodoo, we conjure helpful spirits to assist in our daily lives and spiritual work as well. Whatever path you follow, you might like to appeal to Iemanja during one of your visits to the seashore this summer. If so, try this:

Begin this work just before midnight on a waxing moon. Go to the seaside carrying talcum powder, a light blue and a white candle, rum, fragrant flowers (lily, gardenia, rose stock, or jasmine), a cigar or pure tobacco (with a charcoal block to heat it), a large seashell, and matches in a basket or bag. Light the charcoal block and place it inside the seashell (if using tobacco) atop a mound of sand. Quietly make your plea to Iemanja as you light the cigar or tobacco and candles. Arrange these items on the sand. Sprinkle some of the talcum powder in a protective white circle around the seashell, candles, and smoldering cigar (or tobacco). Pour some of the rum on the ground inside the circle. Cast the flowers out to sea. Sprinkle the talcum powder on the foam of the sea as well—all the while imagining that you are powdering the spirit of Iemanja. Sit down, gaze upon the fire and smoke, listen and look hard as you breathe deeply; see what messages Iemanja has for you. Another orisha of the Yoruba people connected to love, beauty, refinement, sensuality, and sexuality is Oshun. Here is some work to help you invoke her energy.

Reflecting on Oshun

As we are about to move into the notion of cultivating beauty physically, we would be remiss not to invoke Oshun. This is more of a musing than a practical ritual, although if the opportunity presents itself, go for it! Oshun abides by the riverside, a place rich in African and African American lore. To invoke her spirit and pay homage to her sassy ways, you will need to work with a partner.

1. Begin by setting out a brass or ceramic candleholder.

2. Place a few cinnamon, honey, or orange-scented candles on the candleholder.

3. Light the candles.

4. Gaze into the fire and reflect on the beauty and mystery of Oshun.

In unison, whisper the praise poem:

> Barewa lele (The beautiful one emerges)
> Umale (The spirit-god)
> Arele umawo (One of the family reincarnated)

Repeat until you are both relaxed and comfortable.

1. Spread honey on each other's lips and elsewhere if you'd like.

2. Share the honey between you.

3. See where this leads.

4. Afterward, look around you and see which of Oshun's gifts appeal to you. Collect a few items such as tumbled glass, driftwood, or river rocks. Bring these back to your altar at home.

5. Gaze at these items remembering Oshun is not only goddess of love, sensuality, and sexuality—she is also the protectress of women and children. She is the orisha who is known to alleviate menstrual disorders, help us heal from physical, sexual, or psychological abuse, and increase our fertility—not an orisha to take lightly!

Hydrosols for Intimate Apparel

The summer is a very appropriate time to experiment with hydrosols, washing your intimate apparel, silks, and scarves in the gentle essences of blossoms. Fill a basin ⅔ full of spring water. Add ¼ cup soapwort infusion (see shampoos in Spring chapter; soapwort is used traditionally for valuable textiles). Next, add one cup of your favorite hydrosol. Swish clothing in this water gently to work up lather. Soak twenty to thirty minutes. Rinse. Hang up to dry.

Qualities of the three most popular hydrosols to consider:

1. Lavender is relaxing and unisex.

2. Neroli builds confidence in sexuality, and helps with recovery from embarrassment.

3. Rose lends energy, is stimulating, and aids the adventurous spirit.

Bay Rum Cologne

This old-fashioned charmer makes a good Father's Day or graduation gift. It gets better with age, so you can make it in the summer and store it properly, then later give it as a winter holiday gift. Either way, the special man in your life will enjoy the scent, love, and care that goes into this gift.

    20 drops clove bud essential oil
    100 drops bay leaf essential oil
    6 ounces 100-proof vodka or Everclear alcohol, divided
    1 (6-inch) piece of cinnamon
    1 teaspoon whole Jamaican allspice
    4–5 bay leaves
    ⅓ cup pure witch hazel tincture
    1 teaspoon aloe vera

Mix the essential oils with half of the alcohol or vodka. Stir with a stirring rod or swirl. Leave forty-eight hours. Crack the cinnamon stick into small pieces. Crush allspice balls and bay leaves using a mortar and pestle. Add the rest of the vodka. Stir and let set forty-eight hours. Add the witch hazel. Store the mixutre in a dark bottle in a cool, dark location for two to four weeks, swirling bottle daily to avoid separation and settling. Add aloe vera. Strain. If it is too strong, add more witch hazel.

Sunshine Cologne

    ½ cup 100-proof vodka or Everclear
    ¼ cup neroli hydrosol (orange flower water)
    Zest of an orange
    1 teaspoon whole cloves
    1 teaspoon whole allspice
    4 drops bergamot essential oils
    3 drops neroli essential oil
    3 drops sandalwood

Pour vodka and hydrosol into a sterilized wide-mouthed bottle, using a funnel. Add remaining ingredients. Cap; store one to two weeks.

Strain the mixture through a sieve covered with cheesecloth. Pour it back into the bottle. Let it mature three more weeks. If you like, you can decant this into a pretty antique perfume bottle or a spray-topped bottle, as long as the bottle is sterilized. This cologne makes a nice gift and keeps for an entire year without refrigeration.

Rose Garden Dusting Powder

1¼ cup cornstarch
¼ cup baking soda
½ cup dried ground pink rose petals
¼ cup ground dried lemon peel
6 drops attar of roses
4 drops geranium essential oil
4 drops lime essential oil
2 drops lemongrass essential oil

Mix dry ingredients in a nonreactive bowl. Drop in attar and essentials oils, stirring after each addition. Pour into a dusting powder box. Apply with a powder duster. If this type of packaging is unavailable, pour the mixture through a funnel into a shaker-topped powder bottle. Add a few grains of rice to stop ingredients from clumping. Shake on body, bed, or inside shoes or drawers to use.

Gentle Breeze Solid Perfume

¼ cup beeswax pastilles
¼ cup fixed oil (argun, moringa, or grapeseed oil)
1 teaspoon lavender essential oil
½ teaspoon geranium (or rose) essential oil
1 teaspoon patchouli essential oil
¼ teaspoon lime essential oil

Melt the wax on low in a double boiler. Add the fixed oil. Stir. Add the essential oils. Stir slowly with a stirring wand if possible. Let it cool but not solidify. Pour into a four-ounce double-walled jar with a screw top. Dab on pulse points or chakras to use.

CHAPTER FOURTEEN

The Healing Garden

Summer is a wonderful time to grow your own healthful garden. This chapter contains delightful ways of using the gifts from your garden to soothe your soul.

Lavender Honey

Trust me, you'll end up loving this as I do. Lavender honey is comforting, soothing, and helps you relax. The perfect nonalcoholic way to unwind is to add a teaspoon of this to your favorite relaxing tea like chamomile, catnip, or even lavender tea.

Fill a sterilized jar loosely with lavender blossoms and leaves. Pour your favorite type of honey on top. Fill the jar completely. Cover and let steep away from sunlight for six weeks.

Alternate: Rose Honey
Same directions, but replace lavender with fragrant, organic rose petals, making sure the plant itself is disease-free.

Ambrosia Fruit Salad

Though it goes by different names depending on where you are in the African diaspora, fruit salad is a much-loved treat. Inevitably at our barbeques or picnics someone shows up with a tempting salad called ambrosia, or "food of the gods." I have tossed this one together for you, utilizing some of the blessed health foods of the Caribbean, Americas, and Africa.

All fruit should be carefully selected at the peak of its flavor—this takes the most work, for the rest is just peeling, chopping, stirring, and good eating. When shopping, you get hints of the flavor because even when uncut, the fruit should emit a highly aromatic sweetness that is reminiscent of the taste. The color should be rich. Avoid moldy or dried-out fruit. Brown spots on the banana suggest sweetness, yet the skin should still be rather smooth and tight.

½ pineapple (medium sized)
2 mangos
3 bananas
1 extra large watermelon slice
⅔ cup pitted fresh cherries (halved)
⅓ cup plain yogurt (with live cultures)
1 teaspoon orange blossom honey (optional)

Peel the pineapple, mangos, and bananas. Cut the pineapple and mango into cubes. Place them into a bowl. Slice the banana about a half-inch thick and add it to the bowl. Remove seeds from the watermelon. Cube the melon and add it and the cherries to the bowl. Mix the yogurt and honey. Add the yogurt mixture to the fruit. Stir well. Serve chilled.

Melon Tips
Muskmelon, cantaloupe, and honeydew should feel soft near the stem and smell very much like you expect them to taste—these are signs of the melon being ripe and tasty.

Melon Ball and Mint Salad

1 small round sugar baby watermelon
1 muskmelon
1 honeydew melon
1 tablespoon peppermint leaves

Cut the melons in half crosswise. Remove seeds and excess fibers. Scoop out the melon flesh using a small melon ball tool and a twisting motion at the wrist. Add the multicolored balls to a chilled serving bowl. Toss gently to mix. Garnish with thinly chopped fresh peppermint. Serve alone for breakfast or lunch, eat after a main meal as dessert, or enjoy any time of the day as a healthy snack. For a light meal, balance with protein, adding an ice cream scoop size portion of cottage cheese or plain yogurt to half a cup of salad per person. Serves at least four (more depending on the size of the melons).

Sautéed Summer Delight

My mother and Aunt Edith made this basic country dish with produce fresh from their gardens and those of the local farmers to fill in what we didn't grow ourselves. I added the ginger and colorful red pepper because they are healthy and enhance the look as well as the taste of the dish. When you become involved with gardening, it is surprising how very abundant a little patch of earth can be. Sautéed vegetables with lots of tomato are a wonderful way to keep up with the output of your gardens, so nothing goes to waste.

1½ cups okra
1 cup patty pan squash
2 cups tomato
1 green pepper
1 red bell pepper
1 small onion
2 cloves garlic
1 (½-inch) piece of ginger
Cold-pressed olive oil spray or 1½ tablespoon liquid
Sea salt
Freshly ground pepper

Wash the okra, squash, tomato, and peppers. Remove the stems of the okra and cut them into half-inch slices. Remove the stems of the patty pan. Peel and chop the tomato coarsely. Mince the onion, garlic, and the red and green peppers. Heat pan to medium-high. Add olive oil; allow to heat a few minutes. Add the onion and sauté until translucent. Add the ginger. Turn the heat down to medium and cook five minutes. Add the garlic, salt, and pepper; then cook three minutes. Add the okra, patty pan, and tomato; stir. Cover; reduce the heat to medium-low. Braise twenty minutes. Serve as a vegetarian entrée with rice or as a side dish. Serves four to six.

Remembering Ma's Deep Dish Peach Cobbler

Healing sometimes needs to be of the spirit. Sometimes, as in the case of this peach cobbler recipe, food becomes a reservoir, holding experience, memory, and special connections. Many of my people have passed on, but their foods and colorful recipes are an important way of reconnecting with our experiences together.

We'd call this dessert a cobbler. "Cobbler" means many different types of desserts in African American culture, including a deep-dish pie. This one is unusual in the fact that it has a bottom crust. Typically, a deep-dish pie has no bottom crust because they tend to get soggy. This bottom crust is pre-baked at a high temperature, which allows it to keep some of its integrity. It is also baked at a high temperature once all the ingredients are together. We never minded the eccentricity of a deep-dished pie with a bottom crust—we found the bottom crust to taste like a dumpling, which made it irresistible. This pie would never last for two days during our hazy summers on the lake, and it was an excellent way to partake in the wonderful peach harvests from the local orchards. Many areas have wonderful peach orchards. When peaches are in season in your area, try this recipe. You'll be pleasantly surprised. It is comforting, yet a bit different from most peach pies due to its structure and use of spices.

Peach Pie á la Ma

10-12 peaches (from South Jersey or locally grown if possible)
Stockpot two-thirds full of water
2¼ cups plus 4 tablespoons unbleached wheat
    flour (Cerasota or similar type)

½ teaspoon salt

¾ cups vegetable shortening (Crisco type)

6 tablespoons of ice-cold water (keep in fridge until needed)

2 tablespoons freshly squeezed lemon juice

1 cup sugar

½ teaspoon cinnamon*

½ teaspoon nutmeg*

½ stick (¼ cup) salted butter

2 tablespoons whole or 2% milk

2-3 teaspoons sugar

Note on cinnamon and nutmeg: these two spices are incredibly tasty, rich, and feisty if you take the time to buy a whole cinnamon stick and a nutmeg then hand-grind, as we do so frequently in this book, using a mortar and pestle. The spice and lemon perk up what can be a soft, predictable pie. You'll want to be extra-vigilant if you try this approach, however, because in a dessert as delicate as this one, your spices need to be ground ultra-smooth and fine.

Alive and well in my memories, I can still see and hear them (the big and little sisters) in our country kitchen, even as I share this recipe with you.

Preheat oven to 425 degrees Fahrenheit.

Parboil ten to twelve scrubbed, ripe but firm peaches by adding them to a pot of boiling water. Let them boil about three minutes, then remove them from the heat and carefully pour out the hot water. Cover the peaches with cold tap water. Cover and let stand until later.

Put the 2¼ cups of flour in a large bowl. Add the salt. Stir with a whisk to blend. Cut in the shortening a little at a time. Blend your shortening and flour with two cold butter knives 'til nice and crumbly. Take the water out of the refrigerator. Sprinkle one spoon at a time over the flour to moisturize it. Continue to sprinkle the dough with the ice water and mix using just enough for the dough to hold together (don't use too much!).

Make two equal-sized balls from the dough. Roll out one ball at a time on the floured surface (a countertop or large cutting board) 'til about ¼-inch thin, aiming to fill a 9-inch metal pie pan.

Cut two circles from the dough, slightly larger than the pan.

Place one circle of dough in the baking dish and prick it gently with a fork. Pre-bake for five minutes at 425 degrees.

Meanwhile, drain the peaches in a colander. Peel and slice the peaches around the pit, about a half-inch thick (each peach should yield six to eight slices). Use the pits for another project or discard.

Sprinkle the peach slices with the lemon juice.

Mix the cup of sugar, remaining flour, cinnamon, and nutmeg. Coat the peaches with this mixture by sprinkling evenly by hand.

Remove the piecrust from oven.

Cover with peach and seasoning mixture.

Slice the butter thinly, then cut it into tiny cubes. Dot the peaches lightly with this butter.

Cover the pie with the remaining crust.

Crimp the edges to seal; prick the crust with a fork.

Three-fourths of the way through the baking, Aunt Edith, who had her own soul food restaurant for a time, puts her hands on her ample hips and suggests brushing the top side of the crust with some milk and tossing a little sugar atop the milk. This makes a fine glaze.

Sprinkle a little more sugar chil', then toss you some cinnamon and nutmeg lightly over the milk. Put it way back in the oven; bake 'til golden brown and peaches are bubbly.

Baking time is about one hour. Serve warm with cream or softened vanilla ice cream.

CHAPTER FIFTEEN

Get Juiced

Homemade Juices, Smoothies, and Iced Beverages

The Songhai Way of Health and Beauty

The idea of blending elements of cultivated society with ingredients of a completely wild origin is an ancient concept recorded in the Songhai Empire of ancient Africa. The Songhai see the landscape as filled with numerous spirits living in all aspects of the natural world. They believe these diverse entities can come together for the greater good of humans. As such, the Songhai understand that illnesses and disorders are curable using combinations that bring together wildcrafted and harvested flowers, cultivated roots, stems, and flowers with products associated with farming like milk, cheese, grains, and eggs. A synergy develops by bringing together these disparate elements of nature, which has been found over the centuries to be very healing.

Next you will find several recipes that incorporate the Songhai philosophy. These nurturing formulas are affirming, emollient, softening, and wholesome in a holistic manner.

BENEFITS OF FREEZING FRUIT

Freezing ripe fruit helps save money because foods spoil more quickly during warmer months if you live in a hot, humid area and don't have air-conditioning. Freezing enables you to buy in bulk from food co-ops and prepare the food in advance. The freezer works wonders to enhance smoothies. Chipped ice adds body and a welcomed chill. You can freeze peeled bananas in plastic freezer bags or containers. Freshly picked berries freeze well and add great fiber and fresh taste to smoothies. Peaches and apples should be blanched in boiling water first, then cooled, peeled, cored or pitted, sliced, and then frozen. Keep these on hand so they are ready to whip up into a smoothie when the mood strikes you. Having fruits prepared in the freezer makes it easier to start the morning on a healthy foot, since it is a time when you may feel weaker and lack energy needed for timely food preparation.

Songhai Smoothie

This multipurpose smoothie is fragrant, soothing, emollient, rich, and tasty. Designed for sun-parched skin, it embodies the Songhai way of blending elements of nature. A Songhai Smoothie is enriched by vitamin-imbued strawberries and alpha-hydroxy acid (AHA), an ingredient you'll find in buttermilk. Buttermilk is used in quite a few of these recipes because it nurtures sensitive skin. The emollience of peach flesh and peach kernel oil, creamy coconut milk, soothing chamomile, and relaxing oat straw makes this the perfect health brew. The only problem is whether to drink it or apply it to the body—I suggest a bit of both.

> 1 small ripe peach
> ⅓ cup strawberries
> ½ cup coconut milk
> 1½ cups buttermilk
> 1 bag chamomile tea
> 1 tablespoon cut and sifted oat straw herb

Scrub, peel, and finely chop the peach; reserve the kernel. Wash, pat dry, then chop the strawberries. To begin to release the peach kernel's oil, crush the peach pit with a mallet on a cutting board or in a strong mortar with pestle. Add the crushed pit to a baking dish and add the fruits. Pour milks over the fruit, add the chamomile tea bag and oat straw; stir. Cover; infuse the mixture in an oven set at 170 degrees for two hours. Remove from oven; stir mixture. Pour it through a fine sieve, then press herbal and fruit material resting inside sieve with the back of a spoon to extract healing medicine (careful to keep chamomile teabag intact). Set the sieve aside. Whisk; then pour the liquid back through the sieve and repeat the straining and squeezing process. Dab the smoothie on the face and neck using a cotton ball. Leave for five minutes. Rinse well with cool water. This is a comprehensive treat so there is no need for further treatment. Songhai Smoothie cleanses, tightens, and moisturizes.

Makes sixteen ounces. Use within forty-eight hours.

Alternate Uses:
› Pour this in your bath for a luxurious moisturizing soak.

› Sip smoothie throughout the day, as it is tasty and nutritious.

Salad Crème Facial

When we are out and about during the summer months, people pay a great deal of attention to our skin and complexion. We don't want our skin to appear dull or shiny. This combination of ingredients corrects many skin disorders and sloughs off dull skin. The bleaching action of the buttermilk makes it an especially helpful fading ingredient for unwanted freckles, scars, uneven pigmentation, or discoloration. Alpha-hydroxy acid (AHA)-rich buttermilk gently removes dry skin and an ashy appearance in the process. Buttermilk encourages cell renewal, which slows the appearance of wrinkles, tightens saggy skin, and brightens overall appearance. The lipids in buttermilk attract moisture so your complexion will gain a healthy glow but will not appear greasy. Cucumbers are astringent, further alleviating a tendency toward shiny noses or gleaming foreheads. The North African native plant, lettuce, is excellent for cleansing skin prone to breakouts and acne. Carrots contain healthy doses of vitamins A and E, antioxidants that check aging skin and encourage a youthful glow. You will be amazed, as I have been, to watch your old skin flake off after a few days, replaced by a new layer of rosier skin. Salad Crème Facial is only recommended for combination or oily skin.

2 carrots
½ cucumber
1 cup iceberg lettuce
2 cups buttermilk

Set the oven at 170 degrees. Scrub the carrots and cucumber; rinse them and the lettuce. Spin the lettuce to remove debris and excess moisture. Peel the carrots and cucumber.

Cut the cucumber in half; scoop out the seeds and discard them. Shred the vegetables including the lettuce by hand or in a food processor, then add them to an ovenproof bowl or baking pan. Cover with the buttermilk. Steep two hours, stirring occasionally. Drain by pouring through a sieve placed over a catch bowl. Pour this Salad Crème Facial through a funnel into a sterilized cobalt or brown bottle. Cap. Store in a refrigerator. To use, pour a small portion of the crème on a cotton ball or square. Dampen face with the soaked cotton. Leave on for three to five minutes. Rinse with cool water; pat lightly with a towel to dry. Use this instead of soap, in the morning and at night. Makes approximately twelve ounces.

Shelf life: one week refrigerated.

PEELING THE MANGO

Mango is a healthful fruit that has been incorporated into African, American, and Caribbean cuisine. Peeling proves difficult until one learns how. To peel, hold the fruit perpendicular, with the narrow end pressed to a cutting board. With a very sharp knife, cut with the grain of the fruit, removing the peeling.

Continue to turn the fruit until it is peeled all the way around. Cut ¼-inch pieces of the fruit off at a time, placing them into a fruit bowl. At the center will be a pit that can be discarded. Sliced mango is an excellent food for a brown bag lunch because it provides a surge of energy and it is also very tasty.

Three in One Recipe: Island Laasi

When enslaved Africans were freed in the Caribbean, there was still a demand for a very inexpensive labor force. Many of the colonizers began to import indentured servants from areas they had colonized in Asia. Thousands of Indians were brought to the islands and with them many distinctive dishes of African, European, and East Indian traditions, which merged into what is now considered Caribbean cuisine. Island laasi is inspired by the East Indian drink, mango laasi, which serves as a cooling companion to spicy foods and a smooth backdrop to complex spices. It is a cooling fusion of dairy products and fruit, which fits into the Songhai way of health and beauty explored at the beginning of this chapter as well.

I developed this recipe to be adaptable for hair and skin care. It detangles, moisturizes, and smooths rough ends. The enzymes of fresh mango are softening. Lemon adds shine. If you decide to use the essential oils, they will leave traces of an alluring aroma. Cardamom, one of my favorite pods, is earthy, unique, and spicy; peppermint is lively, green, and stimulating to the scalp. Both must be used in moderation to avoid irritation.

1 ripe mango, peeled
Juice of ½ lemon
½ cup whole milk yogurt
4 drops cardamom essential oil
4 drops peppermint essential oil

Slice the mango as described in the "Peeling the Mango" sidebar. Add it to a blender. Add the juice of the lemon and the yogurt. Blend on medium for about one minute or until smooth. Pour through a fine sieve over a nonreactive bowl. Drop in the essential oils; mix well. After shampooing, pour over hair, covering all strands well. Massage and rinse well.

Alternate Uses

1. Double the recipe. Use half as a conditioner and the other half for a moisturizing bath.

2. As a beverage, follow all directions, being careful to omit essential oils. Chill and drink as an appetizer, dessert, or breakfast drink.

Makes approximately six ounces or twelve ounces when used for hair and bath. Shelf life: twenty-four hours refrigerated.

Healthy Nails

Wash your hands. Rub the tips with lemon to naturally whiten. Soak your clean fingertips in warm soymilk for ten minutes. Wash. Rub cuticles with a full-bodied nutritious (earthy) oil, for example, baobab or cocoa butter (or lanolin gently warmed in the microwave for fifteen to twenty seconds or in the palm of your hands). Rest your hands on a washcloth; let your nails soak in the oils for an additional ten minutes.

Sugar Foot Scrub

The sugar, corn, and flaxseed meal in this recipe sloughs off dead skin. The AHA of the buttermilk encourages vibrant new skin growth, making this a great way to get feet in sandal shape for summer. The combination of sandalwood and neroli delights the senses and tones the skin while providing a tantalizing scent to the scrub. Baobab oil has a superior moisturizing ability.

½ cup sugar
¼ cup yellow corn meal
2 tablespoons flaxseed meal
3 tablespoons buttermilk

1 tablespoon baobab oil

5 drops sandalwood

3 drops neroli

Add ingredients one at a time to a bowl. Stir to moisten the ingredients with the milk and oil. Slather on soles, tops of feet, and between the toes. Scrub gently. Rinse well. Apply black cocoa butter or shea butter to extra-dry feet afterward, or a lighter oil such as sweet almond oil, argan, or baobab for normal skin to seal in moisture.

PRODUCE TIP

For optimal health benefits, use organic vegetables and fruits from your garden or your community. Supporting local farmers keeps your community healthy as a whole. Make sure the produce is very clean. When I use non-organic produce, I scrub it with biodegradable liquid soap and rinse well to remove any residue.

Let's get started by juicing some of the six most accessible types of produce, which also produce good amounts of juice:

Carrots—the antioxidant wonder child. Typically inexpensive and easy to grow, carrots yield a beautiful, sunny orange-colored juice with a rich yet exceedingly sweet taste.

Cucumber—very easy to juice. Scrub the skin, cut in half lengthwise, and juice the entire vegetable. Nice for early morning; good combined with other fruits and vegetables.

Celery—fiber-rich, nice, crisp, bright taste. Good to add to tomato, cucumber, and carrot for salad in a glass.

Pear—juices well, very sweet, great alone or added to other, less-tasty fruits and vegetable juices.

Tomato—because of all the water it contains, lutein-rich tomato yields a great deal of juice. Tomato juice is invigorating, especially when combined with a little hot sauce, ginger, or garlic.

Apple—as with most fruits, it makes a sweet juice that children love. Experiment with all of the different types of apples available during the summer and fall months.

> Fresh herbs such as parsley, oregano, and peppermint (leaves, not stem), and green watercress work well added in small portions to vegetable juice blends.

Juicing

Once upon a time, juicers were rare in the home, thought to be too expensive, cumbersome, and difficult to clean. No more! Today juicers start at well below a hundred dollars and come with just a few removable, easy-to-clean parts. I received one for my birthday and find it indispensable. There are books and articles featuring fancy juicing recipes. I am supplying a few simple ideas here.

Vegetable 8 Drink

    4 plum tomatoes
    2 carrots
    2 stalks celery
    ½ cucumber (sliced lengthwise)
    ¼ beet
    1 tablespoon watercress
    1 tablespoon chopped parsley
    ¼ cup washed spinach
    1 clove garlic (optional)
    ½-inch peeled ginger (optional)
    ¼ teaspoon dried cayenne pepper or freshly ground black pepper (optional)
    Salt or lemon juice to taste (optional)

Juice the first five ingredients one at a time. Roll together the watercress, parsley, and spinach; push through juicer. Optional: add a clove of garlic or ½-inch peeled ginger for zip. For spicy taste, add ¼ teaspoon dried cayenne pepper or freshly ground black pepper. To brighten tastes, add the juice of a lemon wedge instead of salt.

Smoothie

Smoothie is a name for puréed fruits, though you can do the same to some vegetables. The beverage combines liquid such as orange juice, apple juice, or water with pieces of chopped up fruit; some people also add dairy such as milk or yogurt. You'll notice certain fruits are missing from the juicing list, though some of them are juicy: watermelon and other melons, banana, mango, peach, pineapple, blueberries, raspberries, and strawberries. Wonder why? Soft fruits and vegetables make out better in the blender than the average juicer. Juiced, they would most likely get wasted, caught up in the fiber filters, rendering very little juice. (The exception is if you have an industrial grade juicer—some of them can juice just about anything.)

I like to mix soft fruits with ice cubes and juice (orange, grape, or apple) in the blender to make a basic smoothie. Then if I have lots of energy left, I'll juice some apple or pear, and add that to the smoothie as it is being blended. Another good approach is to skip the ice cubes and instead use frozen fruit like berries, bananas, or peaches. This adds more concentrated flavor and makes the drink very cool and refreshing. You can add honey and fiber (finely ground flaxseed meal or wheat germ) to smoothies. On the islands, Puerto Rican rum is often added to pineapple juice-based smoothies to make daiquiris, pina coladas, and other alcoholic beverages. Experimentation is fun and yields surprising results!

Bahama Mama

½ cup coconut milk
½ cup guava juice
1 frozen banana
1 cup pineapple

Add ingredients to a blender. Blend on medium-low for fifteen seconds, on medium-high for fifteen seconds, and on high setting for ten seconds. Drink immediately. Makes two eight ounce servings.

Sofrito

Puréed raw vegetables, fruits, and herbs make this practical yet tasty sauce used in Puerto Rico and elsewhere in the diaspora. I add sofrito to basic stock for hearty bean dishes, flavorful rice, and unique pasta sauces. Sofrito also provides a way to amplify tastes in otherwise bland soups and stews.

1 sweet Vidalia onion

1 red bell pepper (or red aji dulce pepper, if available)

1 orange bell pepper (or orange or yellow aji dulce pepper, if available)

1 green bell pepper (or green aji dulce pepper, if available)

1 banana pepper

¼ jalapeno pepper

4 cloves garlic

1 cup cilantro

½ cup recao leaves (if you can't find these at your botanica or
    local market just add an extra ½ cup cilantro to recipe)

2 beefsteak tomatoes or 5 plum tomatoes

Pinch of sea salt

Dash of freshly ground black pepper

Peel the onion. Wash the peppers; remove the seeds and core. Peel the garlic. Wash and spin the cilantro and recao in a salad spinner. Scrub the tomatoes. Add all the ingredients to a blender. Purée until smooth. Use as a sauce, add to stock, or use with rice, bean, or pasta dishes. It freezes fine in a plastic bag or container. Smaller portions can be frozen in ice cube trays and used in smaller increments as needed.

Juice and Smoothie Additives

› You can enhance these juices, increasing their antibacterial properties, by adding honey, which also sweetens the blend. Other bee substances, including royal jelly and bee propolis, can be added to juices for health benefits.

› A teaspoon or two of maple syrup can be added as a sweetener.

› Spirulina and ground kelp (explored in chapter 10) are a favorite addition to vegetable juices.

› A clove of garlic, onion, or bit of ginger, as I've mentioned, adds energy and immunity boosting power.

› Black pepper and cayenne pepper add warming power and energy, especially useful for vegetable juices with a dash of sea salt.

> › Ground flaxseed adds vitamins, minerals, and fiber.

> › Wheat germ adds fiber.

> › A variety of cold, pressed oils have additional phytonutrients.

> › I recommend borage or evening primrose oils for women transitioning into menopause; pumpkin seed and rosehip seed oil for those who suffer with acne and breakouts; hempseed, flaxseed, or olive oil for just about anyone working to improve their health.

Ice Fun

We like to cool off in the summer. Frequently iced drinks pave the way. Let's have some fun with ice:

1. Buy ice trays with heart, flower, star, or other shapes.

2. If you grow herbs that grow in profusion, like peppermint, sage, rosemary, oregano, lemon verbena, and lavender, you know that you need to pinch the plant back frequently so that it doesn't flower. Flowered herbs are not as flavorful or rich and the leaves don't have as much of the medicinal content. You can preserve summer herbs in ice cube trays quite easily. Pinch back. Wash. Tamp dry with a paper towel. Chop finely. Place in ice cube holder. Cover with a bit of spring water. This can later be dropped into broths, soups, stews, and sauces.

3. Add small, organic, edible flowers to water, freeze, and add to drinks. This adds a poetic, romantic feel to an otherwise ordinary drink. Edible flowers include violets, rose petals, and wonderful bright orange nasturtiums.

4. Icing tea. The secret to good iced tea is picking flavorful, fresh tea leaves and being very patient. Out of the numerous herbs discussed in this book I recommend the South African honey bush or rooibos, the American/Caribbean

hibiscus, peppermint, or rose hips, with or without the addition of quality black tea. Dried herbs give off more concentrated flavor and medicinal content than fresh herb leaf. Use more of the tea than you would if drinking it hot, as it will be diluted later by the ice. Let tea steep and cool for at least fifteen minutes. If honey is desired, add it while the tea is still very hot. You don't need any sweetener with the South African bush teas. When the tea is completely cooled, strain and serve over ice.

Soursop Ice Cream

I first tasted this in Australia on an exotic fruit tour. It is heavenly, and really soursop itself tastes like ice cream eaten as it is. These ingredients come together to enhance the soursop's natural creamy taste with a hint of tartness from the lime and a dash of ginger for spice; you'll find yourself returning for more of this uncommon dessert.

1 soursop
¼ cup water
Juice of ½ lime
½ teaspoon vanilla extract
1 tablespoon sugar
1 (14-ounce) can condensed milk
½ teaspoon ground ginger (powder)

Peel the soursop and remove the seeds. Press soursop flesh through a fine sieve over a bowl. Add water to the soursop. Place this in a blender. Add lime juice, vanilla, sugar, condensed milk, and ginger. Blend for twenty seconds. Pour this into a conventional ice cream freezer following manufacturer's directions, or enjoy as a frozen dessert by freezing in a standard ice cube tray. Makes one quart.

Cucumber Water
Easy and cool for a hot summer day, no need to say more. Try it—you are sure to enjoy its simplicity.

1 English or hydroponically grown cucumber
½ gallon spring water

Scrub and slice cucumber thinly. Put in a pitcher. Add the spring water. Put in the refrigerator for at least one hour before drinking.

Alternate Waters

You can replace the cucumber with thinly sliced lemon or lime for a zesty water—skip the sugar; our system benefits from small additions of acids to the diet. This type of water is preferred for those beginning or ending a fast and is recommended as a way to deter sinus build-up.

Ginger Beer

This inexpensive, spicy drink is enjoyed in West Africa and the diaspora, particularly in Jamaica. I like to do this slowly, beginning in the early morning. The drink has the opportunity to brew slowly and the complex flavors meld well if cooked slowly in a Crock-Pot. Those without this tool can use the oven on the lowest possible setting and steep in a covered pot.

2 (4-inch) ginger roots
6 cups boiling water
Juice of lemon or lime
⅔ cup sugar (Monk's Fruit Sweetener to taste)
1 6-inch cinnamon stick broken in half
A few whole cloves

Wash and peel the ginger roots. Grind the ginger root in a food processor, blender (add ¼ cup water to blender first), or pound it with a mortar and pestle. Put the ginger in a Crock-Pot. Pour boiling water over the pulp. Cover, heat on high setting for two hours. Strain to remove pulp; mix in lemon or lime juice, sugar, and spices. Brew in the Crock-Pot another couple of hours. Strain again. Serve over ice. Dilute with water if desired.

Autumn

CHAPTER SIXTEEN

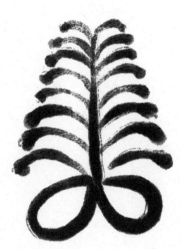

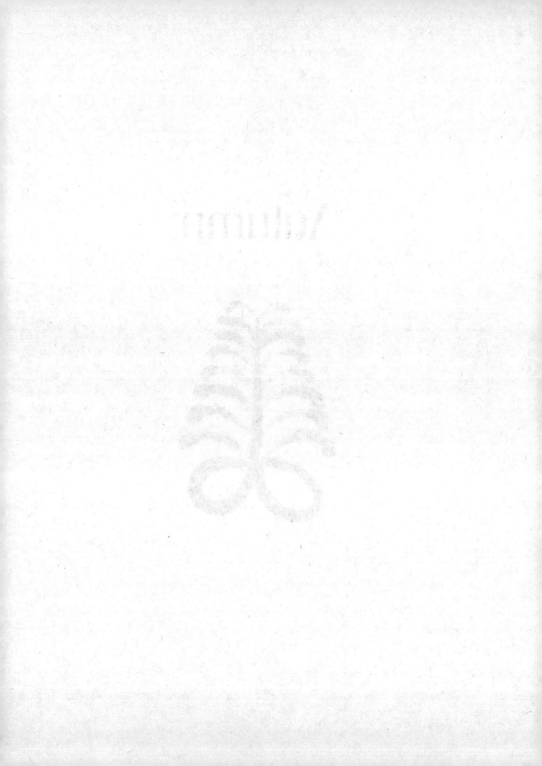

Harvest

Spirits of Fall

Autumn has always been an inspirational time for me as a painter and writer. Warm-colored leaves take flight, performing an ephemeral modern dance across a curtain of cool blue sky. Beneath the curtain, dramas are played out in the heavens, and these have been preserved by the griot in various mythic tales. Not only is the fall a season for revisiting myths and legends, it is a very magickal time of the year. Apart from the sparkle in the air, fall inspires creativity and it is the season for reflection and divination. This is a season when we can set aside time to look upward and examine the messages held behind the veil that separates spirits, ancestors, and humans. In the busy season—that is, the prelude to the "holidays"—it is easy to forget the nature spirits and ancestors. Autumn is a designated time to remember those who have journeyed to the great beyond.

No, I am not stepping out onto a limb here. Look around you each fall and what do you see? Images of graveyards, ghosts, cobwebs, fortunetellers, sorcerers, witches, and decay—people dressed as though they have traveled through various parts of history, different spaces, and distant places. Let's face it—autumn is one of the most mysterious, spiritual, and mystical seasons of the year.

In a mundane way, we as humans seem to be collectively aware that autumn is a time of change. Flickering leaves become a metaphor for the dynamic quality of the ever-changing characteristics of life. We know that it won't be long until Mother Earth's palette shifts from fiery red-orange to the cooler side of the color wheel dominated by gray, blue, brown, and black. Not long till that time when trees are stripped to their bones and birds leave for warmer climes.

In our region, this season of quiet austerity lasts for many a moon. Personally, autumn is also a time of reflection and continued mourning. It is the season when I lost one of the brightest lights in my life. My mother loved autumn. In fact, hours before she died, she was busy taking photographs of the trees across the lake from her home, hoping perhaps to inspire a painting by me.

This is a bittersweet time. We are blessed with the harvest of ripe fruits and vegetables, the air is electric with fiery orange, red, and yellow leaves, but sadly our days grow shorter. Fall is the time to begin the journey inward, into ourselves and into our homes. Fittingly, we celebrate Thanksgiving for our wonderful blessings, a beautiful harvest celebration derived from cultural sharing between Native Americans, European Americans, and African Americans. Today, everyone contributes a bit of his or her own traditions to the celebration, making it a truly multicultural experience. Many people also observe the advent of fall through celebrations like the autumn equinox and Samhain or All Hallows' Eve—ancient nature-based observances that mark the passage of the seasons with an awareness of the cyclical aspects of all forms of life. Across Africa there are a number of cultural observances that also salute the harvest.

Nighty Night Sleeping Potion
Early fall is a flurry of activity. It is an unofficial New Year, with back-to-school being a peculiar type of holiday all its own. Back-to-school carries over to businesses in many different ways, and whether you are in school, have children or not, this time of the year becomes a new beginning for all. Ironically, the animistic-based agrarian cultures that patterned their yearly calendar after the harvest seasons placed New Year at the end of fall, not in early winter as our New Year is currently.

With the winds of change blowing, and holidays upon holidays piling up, autumn becomes a very stressful time. In many ways it is visually disorienting as the world around you becomes noticeably different each day during the height of fall. Amid the flurry of activities, desire sets in (particularly by those of us in the temperate zones) to get things finished before winter or before the holidays arrive.

We become increasingly overwhelmed trying to squeeze so much activity in. We get little sleep, especially not high-quality sleep. I heard of this folk remedy from a doctor who frequently visits Jamaica's highlands. It helps offer some solace and it also ensures a peaceful night of sleep. This Jamaican brew takes advantage of the calming quality of warmed milk and the exotic cardamom pod. You can add a shot of rum to this simple sleeping potion or take it straight.

Take one white cardamom pod for each person and grind it using a mortar and pestle—this releases its medicine. Remove and discard the large parts of the husk. Add crushed pods to a clean cauldron or pot. Add a cup of milk (cow's milk or goat's milk, soy milk is okay, too) for each person. Warm this brew but do not boil. Strain to remove cardamom. Add ⅛ teaspoon vanilla extract. Pour into cups. Sprinkle the top with nutmeg, another spice with a tranquilizing effect on the nerves. Before you know it, you'll all be nodding off to a sound night of sleep.

Los Días de los Muertos

In Chicago, the traditions of Mexico are especially alive and omnipresent during the autumn. In the Pilsen neighborhood where I once lived, I became well versed in the observation of Los Días de los Muertos ("The Days of the Dead"), an ancestral celebration that lasts for several days. I love its specificity, because after all, the departed are not a blanketed group—those who have passed on are separated by age, circumstance, and their relationship to us. Those of you wanting more ways to celebrate the lives of the departed may find these specific Days of the Dead useful:

> › October 27: Spirits without any family or friends are treated
>   to jugs of water (hung outdoors) and pieces of bread placed
>   outdoors to feed their hungry souls.

> October 28: is for those who met with an untimely death, including those who were killed in accidents or slain. These sometimes-troubled spirits are feted outside due to the unsettling nature of their passing from life. There is a concern that confused souls may decide to linger in the home if they are invited.

> November 1: (All Saints' Day) honors the soul and spirit of departed children.

> November 2: (All Souls' Day) is a day to affectionately welcome the spirits of departed adults.

This collective group of ancestral celebrations might help you heal the sorrow of loss through active engagement, festivities, and remembrance. Some of the traditional ways of feting the ancestors are to create organized offerings called *las ofrendenas* for your loved ones.

> Las Ofrendenas: commemorative flowers used as offerings, including marigolds, cockscombs and baby's breath.

> Strewing: tossing flower petals about in the same manner you would toss confetti or flowers during a wedding ceremony. Strewing brightly colored calendula (marigold) petals leading down the path to your door (or if you live in an apartment, you can strew petals from one space in your home to another). This practice welcomes the ancestors and with them, good luck.

> Altars: a space set aside that takes on the air of the sacred. Altars typically contain special or symbolic objects—waters, flowers, candies, fruit, photographs, and candles are favorites.

All Saints' Day Altar
Parents expect their children to outlive them; sadly, this is not always the case. For all those who love their departed children, nieces, nephews, grandchildren, or young friends, All Saints' Day provides a day of remembrance.

1. Dress a table with a pretty tablecloth that hangs low—almost to the floor.

2. Place your departed loved one's favorite fruits, snacks, and soft drinks on the table.

3. Add to this a fresh pair of pajamas or clothing and a favorite toy.

4. Invite the child's friends to come to the home and play with her toys—thereby keeping her spirit connection in the community alive.

5. Place flowers of a type and color that they would enjoy.

6. If you'd like, you can add a photograph or two and a few candles. Arrange the food, flowers, drinks, and other objects in a visually pleasing way.

7. Invite close friends and family members of the departed to add their touches. Host a dinner party to celebrate, remember, and heal.

Building altars is a very moving autumn activity. It is a tender way to keep your ancestors in your home during the holidays, rather than falling into a depression over their absence.

Awuru Odo

In parts of Nigeria the Yoruba people celebrate *Awuru Odo*, a biennial celebration akin to Los Días de los Muertos in Mexico. Many traditional cultures that have maintained elements of earth-based spirituality celebrate and remember the ancestors in a lively, interactive way. The departed are not relegated to an isolated cemetery, instead they are invited to be a part of the family's daily life.

Thanksgiving affords a wonderful opportunity for engagement with the ancestors in this manner. Try setting a special place setting, with food and drink. Prepare specific favorite foods for loved ones, and then leave an empty chair as an invitation for the departed spirit to join the meal.

Another way to face the season head-on is using meditation, botanicals, and centering techniques such as this:

Autumnal Grounding and Centering: a Shea Namaskara Mudra Meditation

A replenishing practice I developed was dictated by the shea butter itself. Shea requires body heat (or some other form of heat) to be used. You may find that taking a little time out to reflect, meditate, or pray while melting your shea is a way to combine plants and spirituality daily. This meditation is also an excellent way to ground and center during autumn.

Sit down in a comfortable position. As someone who enjoys yoga, I do the *padma asana*; those of you who practice yoga might find it natural to sit this way as well (legs folded and flat to the floor). Scoop out a quarter-size amount of shea butter. Place into your receptive hand, then put your dominant hand on top. Now bring the hands together to your chest, squeezing them together. In the Buddhist faith this is called *namaskara mudra* ("The Gesture of Prayer"). Mudras are symbolic hand gestures often shown in Buddha imagery. I like to do the namaskara mudra while warming my shea butter because it reminds me to be thankful to those who processed the precious healing butter so that I can use it. I also think about what power is held in the hands as I warm the oil in my palms, reflecting and hoping my hands will make a difference in this world. To try a shea mudra meditation:

Close your eyes. Take deep cleansing breaths. Scoop out some shea. Put your hands together, bring them overhead pressed together, and then slowly down the path of your center stopping at your chest. Rub your hands together, gently and slowly, to encourage the butter to melt. Concentrate on your breathing, your hands, and your thoughts, as well as the affirmation or prayer if using. As an affirmation, try this: *I am whole, I am sound, I am free to give with these hands in the name of spirit.*

Do this type of reflection for about five minutes a day, to release anxiety, stress, and insecurity. When you are finished, use the shea as an emollient body treatment, rubbing the melted butter on areas that need softening. A ritual involving the moon of the season is also helpful:

Blood Moon Ritual

October's full moon has a vivid name—Blood Moon. Blood Moon is so named because it is the month when hunters have traditionally trapped and killed animals to reserve sustenance for the oncoming winter. For this reason it is sometimes called Hunter's Moon as well. Blood Moon is very fitting because typically the moon of this month turns a rich, blood red. Turning your eyes skyward on a brisk fall evening and observing this particular moon helps you become mindful of stocking up and planning for winter, mentally, physically, and spiritually. It also brings to mind the sacrifices we will all make. This special moon will actually begin as white, but may turn bright orange and then red. Why? It is a moon experiencing a lunar eclipse.

On the eve of the third day of Blood Moon, prepare and ceremoniously pour a libation to celebrate Mother Earth and Father Sky. All participants should wear white (or silver) robes or gowns and jewelry containing carnelian or moonstone with silver accents. The spiritual leader of the groups should clean a chalice with rose water. Dry it. Each member will prick his or her finger with a sterilized needle. Add three drops of each person's blood to the chalice. Pour a cup of red wine into the chalice. Slice a ripe pomegranate in half. The leader squeezes the juice into the chalice. This is more symbolic blood and it also symbolizes fertility. Add a teaspoon of honey. Each member of the circle can energetically stir the potion with a Thet, which is an ancient Egyptian feminine power object, or a wooden wand, if that is what you have available. Go outside. Form a circle holding hands. The leader lifts the chalice, gives humble praise to the auspicious Blood Moon, brings it down, takes a sip, and passes the chalice clockwise around the circle. Each member also toasts Blood Moon.

Harvest Moon

Another moon of autumn is appropriately named Harvest Moon. The Hopi call October's moon *Tuho-asmuya,* or "Month of Harvesting." The Cherokee of the West call it *Duninhdi,* while the Eastern Band of Cherokee named it *nvda tsiyahloha.* Both mean the same thing— Harvest Moon. Sometimes Harvest Moon begins as late as our traditional Thanksgiving. Knowingly or not, most people salute this moon through fellowship with friends and family, and seasonal foods such as cranberries, pomegranates, corn, sweet potato, and other root vegetables. Harvest Moon is also when we count our blessings.

Oya, Orisha of the Winds

Many people are drawn to the seductive ocean orishas Yemaya-Ologun or Oshun who symbolize refinement, sensuality, and fine art. During the fall, my attention turns fully to orisha Oya. Oya is an orisha who cannot be romanticized—she is tough, containing tumultuous energy and awesome physical force. Oya's domain is the cemetery. She is fierce and responsible for swift actions, tornados, storms, quarrels, restlessness, change, and renewal. Oya is the essence of the winds of the four directions—in short, between our delving into the spiritual realm and considering cemeteries and the physical experience of winds, Oya is the orisha of temperate zone autumn. You may wish to engage her energy or at least pay homage during the fall. Here are a few of the particulars about her, useful to know:

1. Her color is reddish brown or rust (rusty nails); she is associated with what are considered "earth tones."

2. She is affiliated with parts of the body including the lungs, bronchial passages, and mucous membranes. She enables foot track magic, magical powders, and magical dust to take effect.

3. She enjoys offerings of red wine, purple grapes, eggplants, plums, chickweed, comfrey, and mullein. Mullein is used as a substitute for graveyard dirt because it is one of her corresponding ewe (herbs). You could also add a bit of chickweed and comfrey to your Oya Ewe Graveyard Dust.

4. Her consort is the thunder orisha Shango. The two guard the cemetery and must be appeased or feted in matters concerning their sacred space.

Oya Altar

Each autumn I toast Oya with her favorite drink, red wine, and build a special altar to her containing corn meal, ears of corn, some tobacco, an animal's horn, beautiful ripe eggplants, and a couple of quirky sweet potatoes. These are displayed outdoors on a simple table where spicy, orange incense featuring crushed orange peel, frankincense, myrrh, and patchouli is burnt in her honor. Next to this, a libation is poured to her consort, Shango. The libation consists of lightning water, which is water gathered during a thunderstorm. Shango also appreciates the tobacco that is included.

Graveyard Dirt

With all the engagement of the *egun* and *ghede* (ancestors), as well as visits to the cemetery, you will need to be attentive to Oya and Shango. You may also desire graveyard dirt, as it is a useful altar material used in spiritual healing work as well as for evil, in which we will not engage in my book. Graveyard dirt is a central component in the Hoodoo's bag of tricks. The lessons of Santeria are especially informative in terms of how to gather and use this ritual dirt. It is gathered from specific gravesites for special reasons:

› Dirt taken from a young child's grave is believed to contain innocence or sweetness.

› The gravesite of an elder who lived a long, happy, generous life supplies dirt with wisdom and compassion.

Elsewhere:

› Dirt is gathered from racetracks, for gambling luck.

› Dirt from a courthouse is used to influence the outcome of a court case.

› Dirt from a foot track of certain animals is used to harness some of their energy.

› Dirt gathered from a specific person's foot track is used to affect that person.

Motherland Ritual

Gather about a cup of fertile soil (potting soil is fine). Put it in a pretty bowl on your altar. Pick out a few ripe gourds and squash of various colors, shapes, textures, and sizes and place them on your altar as well, along with lightning water. If you are not the type to keep an altar, place these items on a nice cloth on your mantel or a windowsill. With this humble rite you are giving thanks for the harvest season while preparing for the challenge of winter. Your preparation has begun early. Blessed Be!

Dirt and Your Physical Health

Mud can be applied to bee stings, an all too common occurrence with the harvest season and with apples fully ripened and flowers in full bloom. Mud, particularly that with a high clay content, can be applied to the sting and will draw the stinger closer to the surface. From there it can be removed with tweezers.

Motherland Facial

> 1½ cups watermelon with seeds (yields some kalahari seed oil)
> 1½ tablespoons rhassoul (earth from the Atlas Mountains of Morocco)
> 1½ teaspoon aloe vera gel

Add all three ingredients to a blender. Purée on medium for fifteen seconds, and medium-high for fifteen seconds. Test consistency. If the mask is too thin, add another teaspoon rhassoul; if too thick, add another ½ teaspoon aloe vera, until the consistency feels right for you.

Apply to the face, neck, chin, and upper chest. Allow mud mask time to set (about a half hour). Then wash it off completely with warm water. Spray face with rose or neroli hydrosol. Moisturize face afterward if desired with an African oil such as sweet almond oil, baobab, or argan.

CHAPTER SEVENTEEN

Soul and Spirit Food

This chapter features an abundance of ways to use the fruits of the harvest. These recipes utilize some of the autumn's most nutritious foods as well as staple foods that offer comfort and solace during the time of seasonal change.

Autumn Fruit Salad

Whether you grow apples yourself or visit a farmers' market, the world seems to be brimming with apples of many shapes, tastes, sizes, and colors each fall. I like to mix and match tastes including Gala, Granny Smith, Strawberry, and Pink Lady to make this salad, also called a Waldorf salad after the hotel in Manhattan. Eating the foods that grow within your village is good for the soul and for the community as a whole. I recommend local produce if at all possible for this recipe.

6 apples, washed, peeled, and cored (squirt with
    lemon juice to retain color if desired)
1 cup dried cranberries
1 cup chopped walnuts
3 stalks celery, cleaned and minced
½ cup yogurt
Honey and ground cinnamon (optional)

Add the first four ingredients one at a time to a large serving bowl. Stir in yogurt until everything is well coated. Sweeten with a drizzle of honey and add a dash of cinnamon for color if desired. This is a salad people of all ages will love!

Apple Cider Vinegar Tonics

Apple cider vinegar was a favorite home remedy of my father and his mother. Here are some of the ways you can try using it:

1. Apple cider vinegar can be taken by the teaspoon three times a day to add energy, aid sluggish digestion, and just to feel good!

2. Vinegar is an excellent multipurpose, biodegradable home cleaner as discussed in the spring cleaning appendix.

3. Vinegar is an excellent skin tonic as well. Try adding ¼ to ½ cup apple cider vinegar to your bath—especially after a workout. Vinegar softens the skin and gets rid of body odors.

4. Diluted vinegar (one tablespoon to six ounces distilled water or hydrosol) revives tired complexions and lifeless hair.

Working with Spices

Okay, I admit it: I am an avid spice lover! These are wonderful contributors to the herbal kingdom, and they are especially beloved in Africa and the Caribbean. In the United States, the use of hearty spices is catching on, especially as we work to reduce salt intake. I say, step out of the ordinary, because after a while it becomes truly boring. I have seen fear and foreboding on the faces of my sisters as they speak of trying anything different in their sweet potato pie or alternate ways of preparing sweet potatoes. The pie is good; the sweet potato is even better on its own. I have used cardamom, one of my favorite spices, in sweet potato pie with great results.

Spices do more than just enhance the taste of food, they also enhance the quality of life. Here are two spice blends that some will consider essential for autumn cooking.

Poultry Rub

¼ cup dried sage leaves
¼ cup dried rosemary leaves
2 teaspoons dried lavender buds
1½ teaspoon multicolored peppercorns
1 teaspoon coarse sea salt

Grind these ingredients until fine in a mortar with a pestle. Store in an airtight plastic or glass container (Ziploc bags do well in a pinch for short periods of time). Label. Rub this over a whole turkey or chicken. You can double or triple this recipe depending on the size of the poultry served.

Autumn Fruit/Vegetable Spice

I find this spice blend useful for enhancing the taste of sweet potatoes, winter squash, sweet potato pie, and spicy gingerbreads. Making these early in the fall sends a wonderful aromatic energy into the air and helps shorten your workload later when this comes in handy—holiday cooking. When you use whole nutmegs, you are getting two herbs in one, as the mace is connected to the shell of the nut. Though nutmegs look like a formidable spice to grind, they are actually quite soft as they are filled with essential oil.

3 nutmegs
2 (6-inch) cinnamon sticks
½ teaspoon cloves
3-4 allspice balls

Grind these ingredients one at a time, breaking cinnamon into smaller pieces first. Use sparingly, as this mixture is very strong and much more effective as a spice than the store-bought type, which is typically quite old, having been on the shelves for months or even years! Store in the same manner as poultry rub.

Rainbow Bean Stew

1 cup each black beans, red beans, pink beans, pinto beans
2 cups sofrito (see recipe page 185)
8 ounces crushed tomatoes
1 teaspoon cold pressed olive oil
1 onion, minced
4 cloves minced garlic
¼ seeded cored banana pepper
½ red sweet pepper
½ chili pepper
½ cup water
1 tablespoon balsamic vinegar
½ teaspoon coarse sea salt
1 teaspoon black peppercorns
1 teaspoon dried rosemary
1½ teaspoon ground cumin
1 teaspoon ginger root powder
1 teaspoon ground turmeric
⅛ teaspoon chipotle pepper

Use canned beans or sort, rinse, and soften dry beans by soaking them overnight. (A quick-cook method can also be used for softening the beans: put them in a pot of about six cups of water. Bring to a boil. Cover. Remove from heat, and soak one hour.) Cook the beans for one and a half hours, rinse, and then use with recipe. Add beans, sofrito, and tomato to a Crock-Pot. Turn on high. Begin heating the oil in a cast iron skillet on medium-high. When the oil is hot, add onion. Cook until translucent. Add the garlic; cook for a few minutes; stir well to mix the flavors. Mince the peppers and add them to the skillet. Sauté about five minutes. Add the water and vinegar. Cover, reduce heat to medium; braise ten minutes. Meanwhile, add salt, pepper, and rosemary to a mortar. Grind with the pestle until fine. Mix in other spices. Stir this into the onion and pepper blend; mix well. After two to three minutes of warming the spices, add this entire blend to the Crock-Pot. Stir well. Cook until warmed through—about two hours. Serve with rice, salad, and corn bread. Serves eight hearty eaters. Feel free to freeze leftovers because this can make several meals for small households.

Pumpkin Soup

2 teaspoons canola or olive oil
1 tablespoon butter
1 minced Vidalia onion
1 teaspoon ground ginger
⅛ teaspoon ground white cardamom
⅛ teaspoon ground cinnamon
½ teaspoon sea salt
½ teaspoon freshly ground white pepper
4 cups chicken broth, divided (see recipe page 228)
3 cups pumpkin purée (canned is fine but make
    sure there are no added spices)
1 cup orange juice with pulp
1 cup half and half
Whole milk yogurt and hulled toasted pumpkin seed for garnish

Heat the oil and butter in a cast iron Dutch oven on medium-high. Add the onion; sauté until translucent. Add the spices; reduce heat to medium. Cook until onions begin to brown. Reduce heat to medium-low. Add one-fourth of the broth, whisk in the pumpkin purée; cover and cook for about twenty minutes. Measure out the rest of the broth, orange juice, and half and half. Add a bit of the pumpkin/onion purée to a blender along with some of each of the liquids; purée and return to the pot. Continue to work in batches until all the pumpkin has been puréed with some of the chicken/orange juice/half and half mix. Once the mixture is all returned to the pot, heat thoroughly on medium-low for about ten minutes. Be careful that ingredients never come to a boil or they will separate. Serve this hot with a dollop of whole milk yogurt and a smattering of hulled toasted pumpkin seeds if desired. This is a filling meal when served with bread.

Roasted Onions with Balsamic Vinegar

This is a savory side dish that goes well with vegetarian casseroles, meats, and roasted vegetables. My mouth waters just thinking about this—savory, sweet, and an autumnal delight!

1 tablespoon olive oil
3 Vidalia onions, peeled and halved
¼ cup aged balsamic vinegar
1 tablespoon brown sugar
Pinch fine sea salt
½ teaspoon freshly ground mixed peppercorns

Preheat oven to 400 degrees. Brush onions with the olive oil and put in shallow baking dish. Cook for ten minutes. Mix vinegar, brown sugar, sea salt, and pepper. Add this mixture to the baking dish. Cook for fifteen more minutes until onions are tender. Eat hot as a side dish.

Corn Bread

1 tablespoon salted butter
¼ cup unbleached wheat flour
¾ cup quality yellow corn meal
2 tablespoons sugar
2 teaspoons baking powder
1 cup 2% milk
¼ cup canola or corn oil
1 organic or free-range egg

Set the oven to 400 degrees. Add butter to a cast iron skillet and put it in the oven as it preheats. Be careful, though, not to let it burn. Mix the dry ingredients. In a separate bowl, whisk together milk, oil, and egg. Stir this into dry ingredients just enough to blend. Swirl butter around in the skillet so it is coated well. The skillet should be very hot. Scrape the corn bread batter into the skillet. Bake twenty minutes or until a broom straw inserted in the center comes out clean. Serve warm with honey, jam, or your other favorite spread. Serves eight.

CHAPTER EIGHTEEN

The Season of Life for Women, Men, and Our Animal Companions

Autumn Season of Life

When humans and other animals enter the autumn season of life, they are what is called middle aged. We all age differently, thus we all hit middle age at diverse points according to our biological clocks. Looking around us at our animal companions, it is easy to see them aging almost at the speed of light, as generally their lives are much shorter than our own.

Middle age is a time when many people first realize the importance of healthy living in connection to the body. Throughout this book, I have shared numerous ideas for using herbs, natural products, and whole foods for optimal health. This chapter takes this book full circle. It is dedicated to autumn, in terms of a life passage, and reviews key features of holistic health, stressing the main points of *African American Magick*.

› Drink adequate fluid—the recommended eight cups of water per day really does wash away some of the potential for illness.

> Eat foods high in antioxidants—these foods are typically brightly colored and include many soul foods such as sweet potatoes, watermelon, collard greens, and other greens.

> Listen to your body. This requires a spiritual connection to signs, symptoms, dreams, and messages that may give you early warning that something is wrong.

> Eat lots of fiber. This prevents waste from stagnating in the body. High fiber foods include oatmeal, flaxseed meal, yams, sweet potatoes, whole grains, and seeds.

> Another way people of African descent have traditionally purged waste from their bodies has been through the use of clay—eating small amounts of dirt. This is thought to bind free radicals and pull them out of the body. The types of clays used are of the purest type available; I suggest bentonite. There is a newer formulation of bentonite that is pleasant-tasting and wholesome, made by a company called Yerba Prima. This type of bentonite and the water it is suspended in has been processed with what they call ultra-purification. Look for it or something similar. If the clay and the water used to dilute it aren't pure, its use is counterproductive.

> Reach out for nuts and legumes just as most of our ancestors have done. Peanut, which is actually a legume, is a healthy, inexpensive, versatile food that is a good source of protein. Black-eyed peas, cowpeas, black beans, limas, and pinto beans—those foods that have time-honored traditions across the African diaspora—are all very nutritious, especially when prepared either vegetarian or using poultry instead of the more traditional pork. Almonds, pecans, and walnuts, among others, are all snacks rich in heart-healthy oils and phytonutrients. The coconut is a large and versatile nut. Cook with it, eat it as a snack, drink coconut milk— getting nutty may end up saving your life!

› Reduce refined sugar, fats, and salt—this is just common sense and can curtail the tendency to develop numerous health problems including the biggies: cancer, heart disease, obesity, and stroke. You can defeat these enemies by eating more whole foods. Love cookies and cakes? How about switching over to more of an emphasis on fresh fruits of the Motherland? In South Jersey we ate lots of melons and tomatoes, just washed and sliced. The Indigenous Africans and Africans in the Caribbean eat plenty of pawpaws, mangos, soursop, bananas, melons, and plantains. These colorful foods are not just pretty to look at, they also satisfy the appetite for a longer time than processed sweets, foods that have been deprived of their ashe.

› Exercise. If you hate to exercise, make it fun. I enjoy dancing, as do many people of color. Dancing is a part of our traditional culture. If dancing isn't for you, think about what it is that you like to do. One of the best forms of exercise is weight-bearing exercise. The weight-bearing exercise most of us do each day is walking. Increasing the distance in small increments yields health benefits and reduces the tendency to pick up excess pounds during midlife. If you are in a wheelchair but can still use your arms, you should also become more active, utilizing your arms to propel the chair. Swimming is another excellent activity useful for folks of most sizes and shapes. It is so gentle that those with rheumatic ailments can benefit, as well as those with various types of physical challenges.

› Consensual sex with a loving partner gives a sense of well-being, self-confidence, and holistic satisfaction. Many people find creative ways to pleasure themselves. It is important to maintain a healthy sex life in midlife and beyond. Widowers, divorcees, and other single people setting out into new relationships should always trust their intuition and spirit when building new relationships and use condoms and other forms of prevention to avoid sexually transmitted diseases, including one of our biggest life threats, HIV/AIDS.

› Be mindful of spiritual health. Traditional African healers, social workers, and psychologists suggest that those who have a sense of community and belonging tend to live a longer, happier life. This goal can be met in a variety of ways—friendship, spiritual fellowship, mentoring, or earth stewardship are a few of the most popular ways of getting involved.

Women's Concerns

At middle age, women notice many changes in their bodies. After the age of forty you should be getting mammograms on a regular basis, unless you are nursing, in which case you should consult your practitioner. Well before that, you should have started breast self-exams.

I am going to spare you the startling statistics concerning disease in women of midlife. I urge you to build on the wise woman knowledge that gut, granny knowledge that you have built on to get you to middle age in terms of your health. Watch, listen, read, meditate, and work hard to stay grounded and centered. Learn to doctor yourself, as has been the way of our people, and if you are very good at it, share this skill with others, particularly those of the younger generation. When you have alarming symptoms, of course, you need to go straight to your alternative practitioner, ND, or MD

Midlife Women and the Four Directions

One of the main reasons there is a parting of the ways in terms of discussing the physical health of women and men is our reproductive organs. This is what largely separates us as humans as well. As our breasts head south, we notice our body continues to evolve and change like the Earth Mother. One of the more challenging aspects of midlife is the rite of passage into cronehood called menopause. For many women, this crossroads begins as early as the forties with what is called peri-menopause—not exactly menopause but headed quite quickly in that direction. Whereas a great deal of health advice is aimed at the physical aspects of a women's midlife, I am stressing more of an African holistic vision using the theme of the crossroads and the four directions that stem from it. Consider the four directions as you consider midlife.

North—Mind and Spirit

As women approach midlife, they begin to really examine their lives and goals, and assess their place within the world as a whole. Many traditional women have children or share in the raising of other children. As these children depart, some women suffer with what is called empty nest syndrome. This is an unsettling time when adjustments must be made for a new direction and path that defines their place in the world. For other women, there may be significant changes at work or with work (when working from home). The new wave is noticeably different—contemporary working women must learn to change, evolve, or move on. Still others begin to examine their romantic relationships or lack thereof. Generally, in midlife, we consider what we have had. Although there is more talk of midlife regarding the body, it is just as important to our well-being to discuss what is going on up north with our mind and spirit.

Recommendations

› Affirmations

› Meditation

› Journaling

› Paying attention to dreams

› Developing or refining interests

These are spiritually sustainable midlife activities, particularly if you have felt that you never had time for such activities in the maiden or mother stages of your life.

East—Looking Ahead

East concerns what we have and what we desire for the rest of our lives. Organizing time and resources so that there is more time to seek pleasure and meaningful activities is important. Taking care of the self has never been more important. As women in society, even those of us who do not raise children, we are usually cast by relatives, the community, or our work environments in a mentoring or nurturing capacity toward others. This is good and bad in terms of getting to know our souls' purpose. Here is what else you can do:

Recommendations

› Do some soul searching.

› Organize and remove clutter.

› Discard or donate physical objects that lack meaning for you.

› Challenge your relationships—work to strengthen, change, or reinforce them.

› Make time for your health—focus on eating well, resting, exercising, and strengthening spiritual connections to the earth or a group.

› Make plans, and work hard to keep them realistic. This might include planning for your finances, your relationships, or for a replenishing vacation or retreat.

South—Reproductive Organs

Women in long-standing relationships may feel a reduced interest in sex that is part physical, mental, and spiritual. This varies according to the situation. Women who have followed a traditional path may feel that their sexuality is of little consequence now that they are no longer of childbearing age. For those who have suffered with infertility while wanting a child, this feeling can become almost too painful to bear. Then there are others who simply no longer feel that their appearance is sexy—this is in large part due to images in the media, movies, and advertising, which often do not include vibrant, middle-aged women.

Last, but certainly not least, are the abundant physical complaints that crop up for some as the result of menopause. The symptoms can include depression, lack of sexual drive, hot flashes, and feeling cold, tired, achy, and irritable. Women in midlife should feel the power they contain and wield it to approach discomfort of the mind, body, and spirit.

Recommendations

› Be proactive, not reactive. Take control, take responsibility, set out to make a change.

› Educate yourself about the mind, body, spirit connection of midlife and well-being.

› Seek healthful foods rich in antioxidants, incorporate home-made juices rich in minerals (featured in chapter 15) and phytonutrients, drink herbal teas with phytoestrogens, and add a whole-food-based multivitamin to your diet.

› Seek out an empathetic, professional health-care provider for regular pap smears, breast exams, annual physicals, or advice about reputable treatments for serious symptoms.

› Make a conscious effort to work at relationships—reading, watching videos, talking with your lover or friends, and learning to love the self you are becoming.

› Stay active. This is a time when exercise of some sort is more critical than ever. Many experts recommend weightlifting (light weights, numerous repetitions in sets of three). I highly recommend this and have found it to be a very effective way to strengthen and tone muscles. Yoga is also recommended for its mind, body, spirit combination, as well as walking.

› Finally, ending on a proactive note, don't feel that you are a victim of your body. Do everything in your power to have the body you have always dreamed of; most likely this is going to involve some type of weight bearing exercise like pushups, sit-ups, or weight training. Perhaps this is the best time of your life to join a gym, start going to the community center, or partner with someone to workout together.

West—Heart Health

Yes, the heart is on the left or west side of your chest. The heart is an organ, yet in ATR it is also so much more. It is the seat of spirit and compassion. It is where we feel sorrow, pain, joy, and love. When once heart disease was more prominently found in men, today women share the burdened heart, making it something we all need to attend to. Since the West is such a loaded territory, particularly for women, there are many ways of tending to it.

Recommendations

› Try to pinpoint what makes you happy and set out to do it. This sounds incredibly simple, yet it may be the single most difficult goal to accomplish.

› Do something good for your heart in a spiritual way. Reach out to your loved ones; don't hold in your feelings, share and express them. This will lighten the heart.

› Laugh—that's right, engage in comedy. Watch funny films, go to a comedy club, buy a book of jokes, and learn the art of joking in a healthy way. Laughing also lightens the heart. Joking, puns, and amusing allegory are hallmarks of African culture.

› Eat heart-healthy foods and drink nutritious juices and the antioxidant-laden herbal teas featured throughout this book. Watch your cooking methods—reach out to braising, roasting, and steaming. Forget about fast food unless it is a prepared salad or smoothie—yes, they are very fast. Otherwise, slow cooking is the way to go. The slow cooking technique preserves nutrients that are cooked away during frying and boiling. A busy person's best friend is a Crock-Pot. As you've noticed, I even make health drinks such as ginger beer in the slow cooker. They are also great tools for those too busy to stand over the stove creating dishes that require enormous amounts of time and effort. Slow cookers just require planning ahead, something I have stressed throughout this book.

› Kick the empty-nest feeling by finding alternate ways of nurturing. During midlife, many women turn to gardening, tending houseplants, window boxes, and if there is the space, a communal or personal garden. This has the added bonus of yielding more wholesome foods and healing herbs that improve your holistic health. Then there is also that spiritual garden I shared in the beginning of this book on pages 24–32. Another way of nurturing is looking out for the elders in the family and the community. Other midlife women give—this doesn't just mean money, though that certainly helps some situations if there is money to spare. Giving can also be in the form of helping the spiritual development of those who are less developed on their spiritual path. Nurturing may take on the form of sharing family lore, community history, cultural folklore, and healing traditions through an apprenticeship program or through community teaching. Some women will take in animals from rescue centers, or feed wildlife like deer, ducks, birds, or even squirrels. Others will develop a very specific animal fancy that leads to raising show animals, while still others will end up striking out on a wild safari in the Motherland. There is no end to nurturing. If nurturing is your way of keeping your heart healthy, it does not need to end after child rearing.

Midlife Men and the Four Directions

I have always been feminine in a traditional way. I loved ballet as a girl. I love flowers to this day and enjoy all that is fragile and delicate about life. I am also very involved in the women's spirituality movement and goddess study, as you may have figured out by now. My ideal life would have been to grow up in a family with lots of sisters and to raise six daughters. This was not the plan of the goddess. Sometimes when you are too much one way, the spirit throws in a curve so that you strike the ever-important (*iwa-pele*) balance through duality. I lived among many males as a girl growing up, and for the longest time I was the only girl in the family. Now my house has many more males than females—even all our animals are male.

In the larger ATR and African-derived spirituality movement, there is attention to the growth and development of manly spirit, too. We see in African communities a type of pervasive negative image of Black males that is more stereotype than truth, and we are acting against that taking root. Those of us truly involved in spiritual development and holistic health must embrace the men in our lives. We must come to grips with the fact that, in some ways, even our beloved women's spirituality movement has short-changed them by excluding them from the new spiritual conversation. Anyone who has suffered gender bias, racial prejudice, or other injustice will realize that exclusion is painful and wrong.

As a mother raising three boys, I know personally that there is a difficult battle when it comes to raising tender, caring, spiritual males in a society that wants them to be thugs, niggas, or at the least, the warriors and providers for the village. I have looked on with great sympathy for little boys who are roughed-up and called men even though in reality they are very early in their development.

Basically, people are people. There are warrior women and men that love to do ballet, cook, and garden—this is the truth but not the cultural understanding. The story of men develops with boys and really with babies, who should be taught to appreciate fragility, nurture delicacies in life, and keep an open heart. Those are the men that benefit society and they are desirable partners.

Basically, most everything I have said about women's four directions goes for men, with few exceptions. Still, this section will go beyond what was offered for the health of women, catering specifically to the holistic development of men.

North—Mind and Spirit

There is a preponderance of spiritual advice and spiritual outlets for women of all ages. The stereotypical image of someone meditating, doing yoga, or attending spiritual services is typically a woman. Men, on the other hand, are cast in leadership roles, leading spiritual and political movements as well as holding leadership positions in the work force. These images are in a constant state of flux, like life itself. As I have said, these are images more than reality, which is far more diverse. Still, being cast in the roles of leader, provider, conqueror, warrior, and boss are taxing jobs for the *ori* (the seat of the north: the mind and spirit).

Recommendations

› Attack stereotypes.

› Are you too shielded to be who you are? What would happen if the armor were to come off?

› Examine what is beneath your shell; visualize it and set it free.

› Is your position who or what you are? Is it a small part of what you are or not you at all? Consider a new introduction for yourself that does not include your occupation.

› Soul searching is an important element of the four directions of midlife. Who are you? What have you always wanted to do? How can you accomplish those things?

East—Looking Ahead

Planning or looking to the east is a very important activity for both men and women. Traditionally men have a tendency to work, fight various battles, and work some more. By midlife, many men question this limited way of traveling through life. Men who carry on through life without facing up to the east sometimes die prematurely in terms of their soul's purpose. It is important for men to make connections, stay connected, and to create and maintain healthy goals throughout life. The midlife crisis that occurs when some men dump their partner who is of the same age for a younger person is often a way of looking back instead of facing the east.

Recommendations

› Assess your life—if it is not as you hoped it would be, set out to make changes.

› Banish stereotypes from your mind, body, and spirit. This might mean changing your physical image.

› You can live longer and happier by being yourself, especially when it is not harmful to anyone, including you.

› Make plans—realistic plans, dreamy plans. Visualize your future—if you can dream it, you can be it!

› You are more than a number. If you want to live a fulfilled, wholesome life, work toward that as you have worked at other things in life.

› Keep your affairs in order, including your finances, health, friendships, and relationships.

› Build toward a happy future.

South—Reproductive Organs

At midlife, men typically get a series of wake-up calls, and many of the messages come from the southern regions of the body (the sexual and reproductive organs), just as they do for women. Men find sexual expression taking a bit longer; they may feel blockages of a mental or physical sort, or irregularity, sluggishness, and impotence. Relief is important. Those who need medicine should seek it out. On the other side of the coin, happiness doesn't just come from a bottle of pills like the commercials for Viagra and other erectile dysfunction products suggest. You can still dance the salsa with your loved one and take long, romantic walks on the beach without pills. In fact, that is just the sort of exercise and sharing to reinforce your holistic health.

I cannot say strongly enough, though, that if you have a serious disease, then of course you need medication. Today, the majority of men do experience some type of prostate problem or another that leads to sexual difficulties and discomfort. Sometimes this suggests an underlying serious illness like prostate cancer.

Recommendations

> An impeccable diet works wonders; eat healthy whole foods from the Americas, the Caribbean, and Africa.

> Include homemade vegetable and fruit juices in your diet. A juicer is an invaluable investment in your health.

> Eat nutritious snacks like nuts, dried fruit, trail mix, and berries.

> Be vigilant about fiber and water intake. Keep toxins and waste from stagnating, as this gives illness the opportunity to take root.

> Learn to trust and listen to your intuition—if something feels wrong, it may well be.

> Build a good relationship with a health professional.

> Be diligent about testing. Test for prostate cancer, and check your cholesterol, stress, and blood pressure—know your real numbers, not just the statistics that defeat your sense of well-being.

> As a preventative, drink herbal teas that build strength, energy, virility, and a strong reproductive system. Highly recommended are saw palmetto for prostate and kola nut for energy.

West—Heart Health

Men's heart health is of major concern, particularly in midlife. Just as I have mentioned in the women's heart section, the heart as a concept has to do with the soul's purpose. Heart, soul, or spirit—however you describe it, it has many needs.

Recommendations

› Men's hearts, like women's hearts, need love.

› Heart is strengthened by conviction.

› The heart maintains health by sharing and being open.

› Heart strength grows when men love others, be it their families, partners, or their communities at large, as well as animal companions.

› Falsely considered more of women's work, men's hearts strengthen through building and maintaining friendship and camaraderie.

› Finding and sharing interests helps to maintain some lightness.

› Stay positive! Negativity is self-defeating and can actually shorten your life. Seek happiness that has nothing to do with money. Spiritually fulfilling happiness is easily within anyone's reach.

› As is true with women, men need to work hard—maybe even harder—to stay grounded and centered. Meditation, yoga, dancing, swimming, and weightlifting can lengthen your life, while also enhancing the quality of your life right now.

› Lighten the heart, go bird watching, fly a kite, or if you have one, take an extra long walk with your dog.

Bones and Joints: Women, Men, and Animal Companions

We have explored the health of men and women using the lesson of the four seasons, the crossroads, and the four directions that are natural to life on earth. Animals are not backdrops to our daily dramas. We all intersect at various crossroads each day. This varies in form depending on where you live, but even in the most urban areas dead and live animals are a part of daily life—dead animals meaning leather, suede, and the meat sold in grocery stores. Though taken from live sheep, wool apparel keeps sheep energy close to our skin.

In African Traditional Religions and African Derived Religions (ADRs), various charms and game hunted for feasts are important aspects of holidays. Live animals are in our homes, zoos, reserves, yards, trees, and conservatories. Birds are the chanteuses that bring joy to many neighborhoods, while squirrels, though pests at times, bring vitality and busy animal spirit to otherwise dry suburban or urban areas. Bees pollinate our flowers . . . and the story of our lives together goes on.

The animals' environment, indoors or out, benefits from the use of whole foods, botanicals, natural products, and the types of biodegradable household cleaners stressed in the spring cleaning section of this book. Moreover, whenever possible and with the permission of your holistic veterinarian, if your animal friend is ill, share some of the herbal teas and whole foods discussed in this book with your animal companions. Introduce whole foods in small amounts if he or she is not used to anything beyond commercial foods.

For the Birds

Many types of birds (both wild and domestic) enjoy fresh fruit, salad greens, certain herbs, honey, nuts, and a few seeds. Seeds should not make up the bulk of a domestic bird's diet as was previously thought; instead, they should be a treat given sparingly. An occasional spray with calming, pure hydrosol such as rose or lavender seems to help an agitated, caged bird settle down.

Our Dog and Cat Friends

Dogs and cats that experience emotional upsets benefit from the very gentle tincture Bach Rescue Remedy, a flower essence that is added to their water—just a few drops will do. There is a whole array of flower essences with very specific qualities to address various emotional challenges in humans, birds, and other animals. I have given my puppy chamomile and peppermint tea to help him settle into our home when he was first adopted. I added just a small amount to his regular drinking water. He is a huge dog, but he loves tiny blueberries added to his meat-based food. Our dog loves large raw bones, as do many others.

Of course, everyone knows cats love catmint, also called catnip. They love some of the other herbs as well, and adore certain fruits like cantaloupe. I have quite a challenge keeping our cats off the cutting board when I am preparing mushrooms or cucumber, of all things. My cats love all things that smell of the forest, especially game. We make an effort to give them appropriately sized raw bones as well as raw meat, and their health shines in return. I do this now, when they are still young, in an effort to help them maintain healthy dispositions, organs, and especially agile joints during what we hope will be a long and happy life.

Use your judgment and patience when introducing new foods to animals, and if the idea overwhelms you, reach out for the newer food formulas that are organic, which contain sunflower seed meal, flaxseed meal, healthy oils, and little grain if any. There are also freeze-dried organic meat-based foods for cats and dogs. These are especially good because they cut down on wasted water and excess packaging, such as discarded cans from canned animal food. The freeze-dried food often contains finely cut bones, which are good for dogs and cats as well. Meat rolls work in much the same way. The food comes in a large roll and you simply peel off the packaging, cut the meat in chunks and serve it to your animal friend. Wild game foods, as well as meat and bone food pre-prepared then sold by numerous suppliers, are other convenient options that offer variety. Online suppliers of holistic products and organic foods come in handy.

Too often we forget that we are simply animals ourselves. Animals of all sorts are important to sustainable life on earth, just as the plants are essential to our ecosystem.

Joints Affect Us All

The lessons of *African American Magick* concern crossroads, particularly the meeting ground of mind, body, and spirit. We have to look at where we came from and realize where we are headed. No one and nothing is exempt from this conversation. We need to learn to live with nature, respecting our mother as she is embodied in the land, and learning our role in a sustainable life on Earth. Every decision made should include a concern for sustainability.

I want to end with our joints because they play such an important role in helping us move forward. "Us" is not human-centric, but includes our animal companions as well as those in the wild. We are all joined together as creatures of this earth.

Through the aging process we become more keenly aware of our joints. With our animal companions, this is noticed much more quickly than in the human life span. With some animals, such as a large dog like our mastiff, joint struggles can begin as early as two years old. In midlife, humans and animals hear creaking and snapping almost as though we need oil. We make jokes about feeling rusty and needing some lubrication.

Wear on the joints is called osteoarthritis, and it is influenced by inflammation. Anti-inflammatory natural foods, especially those with coumarin, alleviate this type of joint discomfort. One of the best natural NSAIDs (nonsteroidal, anti-inflammatory drugs) is ginger—a very popular ingredient in African, American, and Caribbean cooking.

Commercial NSAIDs are making the news these days as some of the manufactured types like Vioxx have met with legal controversy, specifically allegations that use of such drugs may lead to heart attacks and strokes. NSAIDs block the formation of inflammation-inducing substances similar to hormones. Ginger blocks prostaglandins and leukotrienes while also breaking down inflammatory acids within the joints' fluid. Turmeric and cloves also help. (The combination of ginger, turmeric, and cloves is also used to make curried dishes so popular in Jamaican, West African, and Caribbean cuisine.) Frankincense, the beloved East African resin, shows some potential benefits as well. Several companies are busy developing and marketing supplements with natural ingredients that work like pharmaceutical NSAIDs. One company called New Chapter has developed Zyflammend, which combines extracts of ginger and turmeric with other antioxidant, anti-inflammatory herbs. Another company from Europe is bringing together ginger and galangal, two very accessible herbs. Wonder why you have never heard of these pain relievers? These supplements meet with resistance for economic and political reasons—it has been suggested that special interest groups and lobbyists from the pharmaceuticals community block reports on them. You should keep an open mind, cook with these ingredients, and seek out reputable sources of these ingredients prepared as dietary supplements if you are seeking relief using natural sources.

Other ways to reinforce the joints and defeat painful inflammation are food-based. Eating oily fish, a characteristic of African American soul food such as mackerel and salmon, helps a lot, especially when combined with ginger. Other fish that strengthen joints as well as bones include herring, sardines (with the bones), and tuna. Cutting down on omega-6 oils found in corn oil, safflower oil, sunflower oil, and margarine helps. Staying mindful and listening to the body so that you can identify allergy triggers is very helpful as well.

By far, my favorite way of bringing immediate relief to joint pain is stretching. Each and every morning I stretch my back—as soon as I get out of bed and sometimes on the way out of bed. I take minibreaks at the computer to stretch my fingers, arms, and legs. I do the sun salutation from yoga as many times as I can fit in to my day. Most importantly, I also use my body. I dance, garden, walk, and do housework. People who suffer from muscular or bone pain may assume the way to defeat it is to rest and sit still. Nothing could be further from the truth.

Glucosamine and Chondroitin

Two of the newer natural supplements to gain international attention are glucosamine and chondroitin sulfate. They are natural and found in the body. Glucosamine is an amino sugar believed to play a role in cartilage formation and repair—it gives cartilage elasticity. Glucosamine is extracted from seafood tissue. Chondroitin comes from shark cartilage and similar sources.

People report pain relief, and animals also appear to benefit from glucosamine and chondroitin sulfate. For animals it is typically included in their food formula or added to more natural diets as a supplement from a capsule.

According to the Arthritis Foundation, glucosamine and chondroitin sulfate help mild to moderate osteoarthritis.[1] Pain relief similar to that from NSAIDs such as aspirin and ibuprofen is experienced after six to eight weeks of consistent use. If glucosamine-chondroitin sulfate does not provide relief by that point, even after sustained use, chances are it never will, and its use should be suspended.

Recommended Dosage (Arthritis Foundation):

› 1,500 mg glucosamine

› 1,200 mg chondroitin

Used for at least six to eight weeks consistently. The supplements should be obtained from a reputable herbal dealer and should not contain other additives, which can confuse the results.

Side Effects:

› Soft stool

› Gas

Contraindications:

› People taking blood-thinning medications and blot-clotting agents should consult with their health-care professional.

> Those allergic to shellfish may have an adverse reaction, but not always. This requires consultation with a professional as well.

> Diabetics must also check in with their health-care professional because the supplement is a sugar.

Chicken Broth

Scientific tests suggest humble chicken soup lessens the duration and severity of the common cold.[2] The reason is a synergy of ingredients, the most promising of which is the broth. Here is how you can make a low sodium broth on your own.

1 large chicken carcass
8 cups spring water
4-5 carrots (scrubbed)
5 celery stalks (cut in half)
2 small peeled yellow onions (cut in half)
3 scrubbed peeled parsnips
1 cup parsley
Juice of a lemon
1 tablespoon dried rosemary
1 tablespoon dried sage
1 teaspoon coarse sea salt
2 teaspoon freshly ground multicolored peppercorns
3 large dried bay leaves

Put the carcass and water in a stockpot. Add the vegetables, parsley, and lemon juice. Grind the rosemary, sage, sea salt, and peppercorns finely using a mortar and pestle; then add them to the pot along with the bay. Bring up near a boil on medium-high heat. Cover; reduce to medium-low. Simmer for three hours. Remove veggies and bones from the liquid. Let it cool.

This full-bodied tasty broth enhances rice, bean, or vegetable dishes as well as making excellent chicken noodle soup and stews.

BONE CHARM

We talk about our bones in relation to spiritual matters as much as our heart. We feel our intuition in our bones. We feel luck and the oncoming rainstorm in our bones. We feel pain in our bones, and we consider large healthy people to be "big-boned." One of the most famous American lucky charms is the wishbone. Here is a way you can preserve one for your kitchen as an emblem of good luck.

1. Take a wishbone from a turkey (preferably) or a large roasting chicken.

2. Boil this for fifteen minutes.

3. Remove; allow it to cool off.

4. Add the wishbone to a bowl of bleach. Bleach and sanitize it for one hour.

5. Set it out in the sun for further brightening.

6. Hang this up on red ribbon in your kitchen for health and vitality or tuck it into your mojo bag.

Bones of Nature

As we grow older, bones become an increasing concern. We work to avoid broken, brittle, or weakened bones. In various areas of this book, I have hit upon bone-strengthening foods and herbs. Remember to consume calcium-rich foods such as collard, mustard, turnip greens, kale, fish, and dairy products that have sustained people of Africa and African descent for hundreds of years. Vegans or those who are lactose intolerant can still build calcium stores through calcium-rich vegetables as well as the numerous types of alternate milk on the market that are enriched with calcium, including rice milk, soymilk, oat milk, and even almond milk, in addition to fortified orange juice. Health experts advise those building their calcium stores to cut down on alcoholic beverages, caffeine, and foods and drinks high in sodium. Eating soy products like tofu and seitan helps strengthen the bones, as does boron-rich pineapple and peach.

Our avian friends love to forage for organic fruits and vegetables, millet spray, and nuts or seeds given as the occasional treat. Our most common animal companions, cats and dogs, benefit from additions to their diets similar to those enjoyed by humans. Many newer formulas for middle-aged to elderly cats and dogs include ample whole, human-grade foods such as fruits, vegetables, and fibers like flaxseed or sunflower meal. Glucosamine and chondroitin are given as supplements and are sometimes added to the food formula itself. Contemporary breeders and holistic veterinarians stress an animal-specific diet for dogs and cats that is rich in human-grade raw meat or game (no meat by-products) and raw bones appropriate to the breed size and age, as this is what these animals thrive on in the wild. I have tried this with my own animal companions with very good results.

Many dogs develop allergies, and indeed our dog has allergies to corn and wheat, dominant ingredients in many dry foods. This may sound odd, but the two grains actually make his hair fall out in huge patches—not a pretty sight. Our dog, like many others in our community, thrives on a protein-rich, meaty diet with the addition of some blueberries, yogurt, flaxseed meal or oil, glucosamine-chondroitin, garlic, a little ginger, and some olive oil. The most prominent coat conditioner featured in cat and dog health food formulas is avocado meal. Speaking of allergies, olive oil, shea butter, baobab or moringa oil, as well as many of the other wonderful oils from Africa, can be smoothed onto the coat of cats and dogs to reduce human animal-dander allergies.

The human food that dogs, cats, and birds do not tolerate at all is chocolate. It can be deadly, so avoid leaving it around where they can get at it. Onions are dangerous for cats, while parsley is harmful to animals with kidney conditions.[3]

Healthy Teeth, Gums, and Supporting Bones

In middle age, poor dental hygiene built up over the years comes home to roost. Suddenly, yellow teeth from smoking and drinking certain beverages such as coffee and black tea become very apparent. It is possible to use whole foods and herbs for dental hygiene. For example, black tea stains and gradually yellows the teeth because of the high amount of tannins it contains, yet tannins also have many positive functions. Strawberries have a natural bleaching effect, lightening the stains on teeth, as do citrus fruits used in moderation, so as not to strip enamel. Sage leaf from the garden is an easy-to-use tooth freshener—just wiping the leaves across the teeth cleanses. Chewing peppermint leaf freshens the breath. Broad-spectrum cleansing agents in neem, tea tree oil, and myrrh make the trio excellent at fighting gingivitis, an inflammation of the gums, and periodontal disease, a more serious, low-grade bacterial infection of the gums, bones, and ligaments supporting the teeth. The tannins in green tea, bay, eucalyptus, oak, fir, and juniper tighten surrounding tissue and cleanse the teeth, combating many types of gum disease. Chewing various roots and twigs for dental health is a way of life in Africa. Chewing herbs including neem twig, licorice root, and marshmallow root are natural dentifrices. Antibacterial/antiviral agents in echinacea, bloodroot, calendula, lavender, pine, and aloe are helpful at deterring gum disease. Look for toothpastes that contain combinations of these herbal ingredients. Myrrh mouthwash is featured in this book on page 53. Taking a multivitamin helps maintain good teeth throughout life. Vitamins C (ester C) and E in particular play an important role in dental health, as does the antioxidant coenzyme Q10, which is being added to some natural toothpaste formulas.

Finally, don't be taken in by the urban folklore that dry commercial foods cleanse animals' teeth. Ask yourself, does eating a bowl of crunchy cereal in the morning replace brushing your own teeth before setting out into the world? Would you go to school or work that way? I don't think so. Dogs' and cats' overall health benefits from having their teeth brushed at home, as well as from some attention from a veterinarian dentist. Herbs that are used in cleansing the teeth of animals include thyme or parsley tea. Teeth, gums, and the bones that support them need to be kept healthy to ensure quality of life. Periodontal disease frequently leads to serious illness, especially in cats. Moreover, ask yourself if you would enjoy eating every single meal from a box or a can—most likely the answer is no. Why subject your animal companions to inferior foods?

In closing, all animals, including humans, need to have healthy bones, good teeth, quality food, and lots of water. I suggest giving your animal friends purified water or some of your own spring water whenever possible so they consume less toxins.

In the end, whether bird, mammal, or reptile, we are all reduced to bones. We know that Africa is the Motherland of civilization because of the ancient bones that rest in her soils. Understanding the integration of mind, body, and spirit in African holistic health requires that we see ourselves in relation to the environment. No one is too young, old, big, small, or different to embrace a holistic lifestyle.

We end this grimoire and holistic journey through the seasons of life at middle age. I am hoping that building on healthy habits throughout your life will help you and your animal companions live a long, healthy, sustainable life in accord with the earth and her needs that takes you well beyond middle age. It has never been more important to stick together as creatures of the earth, unified with the spirit of environment.

Blessed Be!

Appendix

Spring Cleaning Naturally

Glossary of Natural Home Cleaning Terms

Abrasive: describes an ingredient that uses friction to wear away wax, dirt, grime, and stains in a process called abrasion.

Acidic: describes a compound that readily gives protons to other substances. When dispersed in water, acids conduct electricity. Inorganic (mineral acids) include sulfuric, nitric, hydrochloric, and phosphoric acid. Organic acids include acetic, citric, hydroxyacetic, and oxalic acids. Acids aid in housecleaning by breaking down dirt stains and deposits. They are used for resistant, difficult-to-cleanse projects like cleaning the sink, toilet, and tub, and removing rust, tarnish, and mineral deposits caused by hard water. Natural acids include Tabasco sauce, ketchup, tomatoes, milk, and lemon, orange, or lime juice.

Active ingredients: ingredients designed to achieve the product's objectives.

Aerosol: a substance dispersed by air.

Alkaline: describes solutions with a pH higher than 7, used to strip wax, degrease, or cleanse soil. Alkaline solutions contain more hydroxide ions than hydrogen ions. They react with skin, sometimes causing major irritation or even burns. Sodium hydroxide, potassium hydroxide, and sodium carbonate are strongly alkaline.

Allergenic: describes an irritant or a substance that causes an allergic reaction.

Anhydrous: describes an ingredient or product that has all of its water removed, for example anhydrous lanolin, which is used to make salves and balms to protect or soothe the skin.

Antibacterial: describes ingredients that attack bacteria.

Antibiotic: describes a substance usually made from mold or bacterium that kills micro-organisms that have the potential to infect or cause disease.

Antifungal: describes substances that fight fungi.

Antimicrobial: describes substances that prevent bacterial contamination and the microbial deterioration it allows. Usually small amounts of preservatives are used to perform this function.

Antiseptic: describes ingredients with the property of destroying disease or infection-causing micro-organisms.

Antiviral: describes ingredients that fight viruses.

Biodegradable: describes an ingredient or product with the inherent ability to decompose.

Broad spectrum: describes ingredients with multiple cleansing properties.

Build-up: dense deposits of dirt, grime, or wax.

Calcium carbonate: the chief mineral that causes hard water. It is a combination of chalk and limestone.

Caustic: describes a strong alkaline substance that irritates the skin on contact.

Deodorize: to remove odors.

Detergents: typically synthetic ingredients that work like soap but are more effective at penetrating minerals thereby leaving fewer residues behind.

Disinfectant: an ingredient or process that destroys micro-organisms with the potential to cause disease.

EPA: the Environmental Protection Agency—a government body concerned with environmental safety and pollution.

Essential oils: the aromatic, volatile extracts (essences) of a plant. Oils are extracted using cold pressing or steam distillation.

Neutral cleanser: a cleaner that has a pH between 7 and 9, especially important with waxes because high pH can attack wood and dull wax finishes.

Petroleum-based products: as it sounds, products created from using petroleum, a nonrenewable energy source.

Phosphate: a substance used as a water softener.

Sanitize: to substantially remove undesirable organisms like bacteria, preferably without negatively impacting the wholesome qualities that need to be retained.

Saponin: a natural surfactant with a detergent-like action that is found in plants. The word "saponin" is derived from the soapwort plant (*Saponaria officinalis*) because it has strong foaming and lathering action. Saponins are toxic to some fish because of the type of glycosides they contain. Saponins seem to have antimicrobial and antibiotic properties.

Solvent: a liquid that dissolves other substances. The two most common solvents used in home cleaning are water and alcohol.

Submersion: to soak in a liquid to cleanse.

Surfactant: a substance that lowers the surface tension of water, modifying the wetting, dispersal, foaming, and spreading abilities of a product.

Tarnish: a thin film or residue that changes or dulls the color of metals.

Volatile: describes an element, ingredient, or constituent that evaporates during drying.

Tools for Holistic Home Cleaning

Chamois: a deerskin cloth used for polishing metal and buffing furniture. Availability: can be purchased from automobile supply shops, hardware stores, and art supply shops.

Dust mask: protects respiratory system from fine particles of dust, ground herbs, and resins as well as other materials encountered during product creation and cleaning.

Latex or other protective gloves: protect hands while cleaning.

Rags: pieces of cloth—strong cotton works very well. Uses: for polishing and some cleaning. Availability: recycle and reuse old, clean clothing like t-shirts; purchase cheap clothing from secondhand stores. New rags can be purchased from automobile supply shops, hardware stores, and art supply shops.

Sponge: natural sea sponge or pure cellulose work best. Natural sea sponges are the skeletons of aquatic, lower invertebrate life forms called poriferans. Uses: to spot clean areas all over the house, including floors, bath, basin, toilet, tiles, and appliances. How to use: sponges that are suspected of containing disinfectants can be sterilized with boiling water (submerged in a pan for about five minutes or by washing in a dishwasher). Availability: widely available in grocery stores, health food stores, and hardware shops. Precautions: sponges that say "kills odor" or "disinfects" contain disinfectants, some of which are thought to lead to resistance to antibiotics.

Spout top bottle (squirt bottle): Uses: to store and dispense homemade cleansing products. How to use: shampoo and conditioner bottles can be reused (recycled) by sterilizing first with boiling hot water. Precautions: to avoid confusion, homemade cleanser put in these types of bottles should be labeled like all natural home cleaning products to avoid potential injury or danger. Availability: most people have these types of bottles from shampoo products or dish detergent ready to be sterilized and reused. Specialty soap making and other craft supply shops carry new bottles.

Spray-top bottle: for general cleaning, dispersing liquid ingredients without harming the environment. Availability: some people have these types of bottles from hair care products or dish detergent—ready to be sterilized and reused. Specialty soap making and other craft supply shops carry new spray-top bottles.

Natural Home Cleaning Ingredient List

Animal

Beeswax: a hard wax made by bees. Uses: homemade furniture polish, floor wax, candles, and healing balms and salves. How to use: melt in a double boiler, or for polish, melt with turpentine; add herbal ingredients and fixed oils as directed by a recipe. Availability: purchase from beekeepers (at apiaries), or from candle-making, soap-making, and general art supply shops. Precautions: since it is usually heated, care should be exercised with formulations and adult supervision of children is recommended.

Diatomaceous earth: skeletons of prehistoric algae. Uses: absorbs oil and water—has abrasive qualities. Diatomaceous earth is a very effective nontoxic insecticide. How to use: sprinkle on spot to be cleansed, and scrub with sponge or blot with a rag. Availability: specialty shops and online catalogs. Precautions: though considered nontoxic, diatomaceous earth contains tiny particles that can irritate the lungs and eyes. Safety is important; use a dust mask to protect the respiratory system, and possibly goggles. While this ingredient kills pest bugs that infiltrate the garden and pantry, it can kill the good bugs too, so it should be used with great care and consideration.

Lanolin: oil found in sheep's wool. Sheep are unharmed by removal of lanolin. Uses: included in leather cleaners and used for healing balms as well as salves. How to use: either directly, placed on a rag, or melted in a double boiler to which fixed oils and essential oils are added as per recipe. Availability: beauty supply shops, herb craft shops, and online.

Shellac: a lac is a beetle excretion. While technically this only defines "lac," shellac is the commonly used term to describe the varnish made from it, which is also used as a finishing medium when painting. Uses: furniture sealant is created when mixed with alcohol, which is used as a solvent. How to use: pour a small amount onto a rag. Treat area, rubbing gently. Availability: art suppliers and herb craft suppliers. Precautions: shellac must be used in well-ventilated areas. Gloves protect sensitive skin, and a safety mask limits inhalation of vapors and helps those with respiratory problems.

Fruit

Citrus peel: peels from citrus fruit contain a natural solvent, deodorizer, and pleasant fragrance. Uses: simmered to freshen the air, added to potpourri, added to homemade incense blends along with spices, added to cleansing water as an essential oil for disinfecting and cleaning bathrooms, kitchens, refrigerators and other appliances, floors, and clothing. How to use: dried citrus peel is used in potpourri and air fresheners as well as incense. Fresh peel can be simmered and added to cleansing water. Essential oils are dropped into solutions as directed in recipes.

Grapefruit seed extract: though not registered with the EPA, grapefruit seed extract is a highly touted cleansing aid with antiseptic qualities. How to use: add by the teaspoon as directed to water or other dispersal agents such as vegetable-based soap for cleansing.

Lemon: this fruit is one of the best natural cleaning ingredients. It can be used as an air freshener, it has a slight bleaching action, and it also works as an insecticide (for fleas).

Lime: an aromatic antiseptic used in general household cleaning products and air fresheners.

Orange: an aromatic air freshener and deodorant, used in cleaning formulas, especially furniture and floor preparations.

Tomato: this fruit's acidic nature lends itself to removing or reducing tarnish on certain metals.

Vegetables

Celery: absorbs odors, particularly when rubbed on a cutting board.

Corn meal: used as a soft abrasive to spot clean areas such as bathrooms and kitchens, as well as pots and pans and appliances.

Rhubarb: used for its bleaching action.

Vegetable glycerin: used in cleaning recipes as a stain remover. It is also used in herbal formulae to help oil mix with water when making creams, salves, or balms.

Flowers

Rose, lavender, orange blossom, and other pleasantly scented waters can be used in home cleaning. Rose water, lavender water, or orange blossom water is added to the final rinse of wash to scent clothing. Floral waters are sprayed in the air or set out in bowls to scent and freshen the air.

House Plants

Houseplants are used to enhance air quality. These plants include aloe vera, English ivy (which attacks benzene, a known carcinogen), fig tree (which attacks formaldehyde in the air), and spider plant (also for formaldehyde).

Herbs

Flaxseed oil (linseed oil): used in furniture polishes.

Horsetail (shave grass): is high in silica. It is used to scrub and polish pots and pans, and for general cleaning requiring scrubbing action. Horsetail stems are used like sandpaper—they are abrasive. How to use: rub a handful of dried stems on surfaces, rinse. Wash with vegetable soap if necessary to remove green staining.

Lavender, rosemary, calendula, eucalyptus, juniper, sage, thyme, angelica root, pine, spruce, and fir: can be brewed in water to create a disinfectant solution as a tea using an infusion method. Steep twenty to twenty-five minutes with the top covered; strain. These herbs can also be used as general cleansers alone or in combination with soapwort and essential oils.

Soapwort: an important herb for cleaning because it is high in saponin, making it a natural herb for lathering. Its sudsing action is used in personal care and herbal home cleaning, floor wash, general cleansing, and safe cleansing of fragile or delicate fabrics. A tea is made from the herb to extract the lathering qualities. Many plants contain saponins including yucca, soap tree, papaya, and peach leaf.

Sweet cicely: seeds are crushed and added to linseed oil to make furniture polish.

Almost all herbs lend themselves to natural home cleaning. View the essential oils section below for individual qualities of herbs in cleansing the home.

Essential Oils

Antibiotic Herbs and Essential Oils

Balsam of Peru, bergamot, cinnamon, clove, eucalyptus, eucalyptus lemon, eucalyptus radiata, garlic, German chamomile, hyssop, lavender, lemon, lime, myrtle, niaouli, nutmeg, onion, oregano, patchouli, pine, ravensara, Roman chamomile, sarriette, tea tree, terebinth.

Antifungal Herbs and Essential Oils

Balsam of Peru, eucalyptus lemon, eucalyptus radiata, juniper, lavender, lemon, myrtle, onion, patchouli, pimento, sage, sandalwood, sarriette, savory, tea tree, thyme.

Antiseptic Herbs and Essential Oils

Bay, bergamot, cajeput, camphor, cardamom, cedarwood, celery (domestic and wild), cinnamon, citronella, clary sage, clove, cumin, cypress, elemi, eucalyptus lemon, eucalyptus radiata, garlic, geranium, German chamomile, ginger, hyssop, juniper, lavender, lemon, lemongrass, lime, mandarin, marjoram, myrtle, niaouli, nutmeg, onion, oregano, parsley, patchouli, peppermint, pettigraine, pimento, pine, ravensara, Roman chamomile, rose, rosemary, sage, rose de bois, sandalwood.

Antiviral Herbs and Essential Oils

Citronella, clove, eucalyptus lemon, eucalyptus radiata, garlic, lavender, onion, parsley, ravensara, sandalwood, tea tree, thyme.

Broad Spectrum

Eucalyptus lemon, eucalyptus radiata, lavender, tea tree, thyme.

Note: Pine oil disinfects and deodorizes, but it is a potential allergen so it needs to be used with protective gloves to avoid contact with skin, and used sparingly.

Minerals

Alum: a soft mineral used with acidic substances like vinegar or lemon. Uses: to lift hard water stains. How to use: sprinkle on the spot to be cleaned. Scrub. Rinse.

Baking soda: a common mineral made from soda ash that is slightly alkaline, used for cleaning as a nonabrasive soft scrub and to remove or prevent odors. Uses: cleaning clothing, bathrooms (basin, tub, toilet), refrigerators, and garbage bins. How to use: put in a bowl or sprinkle into areas that need to be cleansed or deodorized like trash cans or drains. Add to wash by the cup after water is already in washing machine to avoid clumping.

Borax: disinfects, deodorizes, and inhibits mold growth. Uses: to clean kitchens, baths, garages, basements, ovens, and other heavily soiled areas. How to use: sprinkle on spots to be cleaned. Scrub. Rinse. Precautions: individuals with sensitive skin or those who are prone to allergic reactions might like to wear protective gloves.

Chalk: a nonabrasive cleaner. Uses: spot whitener. How to use: apply to spots that need whitening, wet slightly, rub, and rinse. Reapply or leave on overnight for tough spots.

Cream of tartar: cleans porcelain, drains, and metals. How to use: disperse in water. Submerge metal; soak for several hours; rinse. Pour directly down the drain and flush with water. Sprinkle on bathroom basins, tubs, or tiles. Scrub. Rinse.

Pumice: aids cleansing action of soaps; absorbs moisture. Uses: an abrasive cleanser for hands, hard metals, and hard water deposits. If using a pumice stone, scrub areas that need to be cleansed. Pumice is also added to hand-cleaning recipes, soaps, and other cleaning solutions in pulverized form, as per recipe. Precautions: it is a strong abrasive—use with care and discretion on skin and within the home to avoid scratching or discoloration.

Salt: non-scratching (to most surfaces) abrasive cleaner with antibacterial qualities. How to use: sprinkle on areas that need to be cleaned. Scrub with sponge or rag. Rinse. Repeat as needed.

Washing soda (caustic soda): is sodium carbonate. It has high alkalinity (around pH 11) and cuts grease. Uses: to clean clothing—removing dirt, oil, and stains—and to neutralize odors. How to use: add to wash during wash cycle after water is added to avoid clumping. Sprinkle directly on areas to be cleaned, especially the kitchen and bath. Precautions: potential irritant to skin; wear gloves, and make sure that clothing washed with this is rinsed very well or it may irritate the skin. Use sparingly for allergic and sensitive individuals.

Miscellaneous

Castile soap: an olive oil-based soap, liquefied and used as a natural soap base in a wide variety of cleansing solutions. Dr. Bronner's is a name-brand Castile soap with multiple purposes. Uses: shampoo, (hand washing) dish detergent, and cloth detergent. How to use: add the suggested amount to shampoo blends, along with fixed oils or essential oils as directed. Castile soap can also be used straight to wash and cleanse the body and home. Special precaution should be taken to remove soap scum or build-up that may occur by following up with a vinegar rinse.

White bread: absorbs odors in the air. Place in the refrigerator or nearby when working with onions.

White vinegar: an acidic natural substance made from a variety of different ingredients during the fermentation process. The acidic action dissolves build-up, removes tarnish from metals and dirt from organic and inorganic substances, and helps clean cloth. White vinegar is good for cleaning refrigerators and pouring down drains to discourage clogs.

Chapter Notes

Chapter 1

1. John Anenechukwu Umeh, *After God is Dibia: Igbo Cosmology, Divination & Sacred Science in Nigeria,* Volume Two (London: Karnak House, 1999), 38.
2. Ann Moura, "Of Shadows and Grimoires, Llewellyn's New Worlds of Mind and Spirit" NW035 (2003): 18.

Chapter 3

1. Richard Westmacott, *African-American Gardens and Yards in the Rural South* (Knoxville: University of Tennessee Press, 1992).
2. Robert Farris Thompson, *Flash of the Spirit* (New York: Vintage, 1983), 135–139.
3. Constance Rodriguez, "Sacred Codes: Ancient Keys for Unlocking Soul Awareness" (unpublished book, 2005). Excerpt used by permission.
4. Richard Westmacott, 79–80.
5. For more information, refer to *Pow Wows, or Long Lost Friend* by J. G. Hohman (Pomeroy, WA: Health Research Publishers, 1971).
6. William E. Grime, "Plants Introduced by the Slaves," in *Ethno-botany of the Black Americans* (Algonac, MI: Reference Publications, Inc., 1979), 19–63.
7. United Plant Savers, P. O. Box 147, Rutland, OH 45775. Tel. (740) 742-3455, *unitedplantsavers.org,* E-mail: office@unitedplantsavers.org.

Chapter 4

1. US Consumer Product Safety Commission, "News from CPSC," release #01-083 (press release, February 14, 2001).

Chapter 5

1. Eve Palmer, *The South African Herbal* (Cape Town, South Africa: Tafelberg Publishers Ltd, 1985), 146.
2. D. J. Cobb, "Red Bush Blessings," in *2005 Herbal Almanac* (St. Paul: Llewellyn Worldwide, 2004), 266–267.
3. Ibid, 267.
4. US Department of Homeland Security, FEMA, "Residential Smoking Fires and Casualties." *Topical Fire Research* Series 5, issue 5 (June 2005): *http://www.usfa.fema.gov.*

Chapter 6

1. Claudette V. Copney, *Jamaican Culture and International Folklore: Superstitions, Beliefs, Dreams, Proverbs and Remedies* (Raleigh, NC: Pentland Press, 1999), 86–88.

Chapter 8

1. Umeh, 115–116.

Chapter 10

1. Valerie Ann Worwood, *The Complete Book of Essential Oils and Aromatherapy* (Novato, CA: New World Library, 1991).
2. Francesco Mastalia and Alfonse Pagano, *Dreads* (New York: Artisan, 1999).
3. Lonnice Brittenum Bonner, *Plaited Glory: For Colored Girls Who've Considered Braids, Locks, and Twists* (New York: Three Rivers Press, 1996).
4. Tulani Kinard, *No More Lye: The African American Woman's Guide to Natural Haircare* (New York: St. Martin's Press, 1997), 9.

Chapter 18

1. Arthritis Foundation, "Glucosamine and Chondroitin Sulfate." June 28, 2002. *http://www.arthritis.org.*
2. Jean Carper, "Fighting the Common Cold," *USA Weekend Magazine,* January 6–8, 1995. *http://www.usaweekend.com.*
3. I recommend the following three books for definitive information on herbal health for your animals, *The Encyclopedia of Natural Pet Care* by C. J. Puotinen (Los Angeles: Keats Publishing, 2000), *Dr. Kidd's Guide to Herbal Dog Care,* and *Dr. Kidd's Guide to Herbal Cat Care* by Randy Kidd, DVM, PhD (Pownal, VT: Storey Publishers, 2000).

Bibliography

Abbiw, Daniel K. *Useful Plants of Ghana: West African Uses of Wild and Cultivated Plants*. London: Intermediate Technology Publications and the Royal Botanic Gardens KEW, 1995.

Amen, Ra Un Nefer. *Metu Neter Vol.1: The Great Oracle of Tehuti and the Egyptian System of Spiral Cultivation*. New York: Kamit Publications, 1990.

Baring, Anne and Jules Cashford. *The Myth of the Goddess: Evolution of an Image*. New York: Penguin Books, 1993.

Berthold-Bond, Annie. *Clean and Green: The Complete Guide to Nontoxic and Environmentally Safe Housekeeping*. Woodstock, NY: Ceres Press, 1994.

Bird, Stephanie Rose. *Sticks, Stones, Roots & Bones: Hoodoo, Mojo & Conjuring with Herbs*. St. Paul, MN: Llewellyn Worldwide, 2004.

Bonner, Lonnice Brittenum. *Plaited Glory: For Colored Girls Who've Considered Braids, Locks, and Twists*. New York: Three Rivers Press, 1996.

Boughman, Arvis Locklear and Loretta O. Oxendine. *Herbal Remedies of the Lumbee Indians*. Jefferson, NC, and London: McFarland and Company, 2003.

Boulos, Loufy. *Medical Plants of North America*. Algonac, MI: Reference Publications, Inc., 1983.

Bremness, Leslie. *The Complete Book of Herbs*. New York: Viking Studio Books, Penguin Putnam, 1994.

Buckley, Anthony D. *Yoruba Medicine*. Brooklyn, NY: Athelia Henrietta Press, Inc. Publishing in the Name of Orunmila, 1997.

Caldecott, Moyra. *Myths of the Sacred Tree*. Rochester, VT: Destiny Books, 1993.

Carper, Jean. *Food—Your Miracle Medicine: How Food Can Prevent and Cure over 100 Symptoms and Problems*. New York: HarperCollins Publishers, Inc., 1993.

Cobb, D. J. "Red Bush Blessings." *2005 Herbal Almanac*. St. Paul, MN: Llewellyn Worldwide, 2005.

Copney, Claudette V. *Jamaican Culture and International Folklore, Superstitions, Beliefs, Dreams, Proverbs, and Remedies*. Raleigh, NC: Pentland Press, 1999.

Courlander, Harold. *A Treasury of Afro-American Folklore*. New York: Marlowe & Co., 1996.

Edwards, Victoria H. *The Aromatherapy Companion: Medicinal Uses/AyurVedic Healing/Body-Care Blends/Perfumes and Scents/Emotional Health and Well-Being*. Pownal, VT: Storey Books, 1999.

Glassman, Sallie Ann. *Vodou Visions: An Encounter with Divine Mystery*. New York: Villard Books, a division of Random House, 2000.

Grime, William E. *Ethno-botany of the Black Americans*. Algonac, MI: Reference Publishers, Inc., 1979.

Harris, Jessica B. *Iron Pots and Wooden Spoons: Africa's Gifts to New World Cooking*. New York: Ballantine Books, 1989.

Hohman, J. G. *Pow Wows, or Long Lost Friend: A Collection of Mysteries and Invaluable Arts and Remedies*. Pomeroy, WA: Health Research Publishers, 1971.

Huttman, Tami, ed. *The Africa News Cookbook: African Cooking for Western Kitchens*. New York and London: Penguin Books and Africa News Service, 1985.

Hyatt, Harry Middleton. *Folklore of Adams County, Illinois: Memoirs of the Alma Egan Hyatt Foundation*. New York: The E. Cabella-French Printing and Publishing Corporation, 1935.

Illes, Judika. *Earth Mother Magic: Ancient Spells for Modern Belles*. Gloucester, MA: Fairwinds Press, 2001.

Joseph, James A., Daniel A. Nadeau, and Anne Underwood. *Color Code: A Revolutionary Eating Plan for Optimum Health*. New York: The Philip Lief Group, Inc., 2002.

Karade, Baba Ifa and J. D. Baldwin. "Pre-historic Nations." *The Handbook of Yoruba Religious Concepts*. Edited by L. Olumide. York Beach, ME: Weiser Books, 1994.

Karenga, Maulana. *Kwanzaa: A Celebration of Family, Community, and Culture*. http://www. officialkwanzaawebsite.org/

Kidd, Randy. *Dr. Kidd's Guide to Herbal Cat Care*. Pownal, VT: Storey Book Publishers, 2000.

——. *Dr. Kidd's Guide to Herbal Dog Care*. Pownal, VT: Storey Book Publishers, 2000.

Kinard, Tulani. *No More Lye: The African American Woman's Guide to Natural Haircare*. New York: St. Martin's Press, 1997.

Klein, Cecelia F. *Gender in Pre-Hispanic America: A Symposium at Dumbarton Oaks, 12 and 13 October 1996*. Washington, DC: Dumbarton Oaks Research Library and Collection, 2001.

Lappé, Frances Moore and Anna Lappé. *Hope's Edge: The Next Diet for a Small Planet*. New York: Jeremy P. Tarcher/Putnam, 2002.

Makinde, M. A. *African Philosophy, Culture, and Traditional Medicine*. Athens, OH: Ohio University Center for International Studies, Africa Series no. 53, 1988.

Manniche, Lise. *An Ancient Egyptian Herbal*. Austin, TX: University of Texas Press, 1989.

Mastalia, Francesco and Alfonse Pagano. *Dreads*. New York: Artisan, 1999.

McIntyre, Anne. *The Complete Woman's Herbal: A Manual of Healing Herbs and Nutrition for Personal Well-being and Family Care*. New York: Henry Holt Books, 1994.

Mitchell, Faith. *Hoodoo Medicine: Gullah Herbal Remedies*. Columbia, SC: Summerhouse Press, 1999.

Moura, Ann. *Grimoire for the Green Witch: A Complete Book of Shadows*. St. Paul, MN: Llewellyn Worldwide, 2003.

——. "Of Shadows and Grimoires." *Llewellyn's New Worlds of Mind and Spirit* NW035 (2003): 18.

Mutwa, Vusamazulu Credo. *Zulu Shaman: Dreams, Prophecies, and Mysteries*. Edited by Stephen Larsen. Rochester, VT: Destiny Books, 1996.

Nommo, Nzingha A. (a.k.a. Jill Patrice Bunton). *African Seeds of Life*. Oak Park, IL: self published, 2002.

Offodile, Buchi. *The Orphan Girl and Other Stories: West African Folktales*. Northampton, MA: Interlink Publishing Group, 2001.

Palmer, Eve. *The South African Herbal*. Cape Town, South Africa: Tafelberg Publishers, Ltd., 1985.

Puotinen, C. J. *The Encyclopedia of Natural Pet Care*. Los Angeles: Keats Publishing, 2000.

Purchon, Nerys. *Nerys Purchon's Handbook of Natural Healing: The Complete Home-Reference Guide*. St. Leonards, New South Wales: Allen & Unwin, 1998.

Rashidi, R. "African Goddesses." *Civilizations* 6:1. New Brunswick & London: Transaction Publishers, 2002.

Riva, Anna. *Magic with Incense and Powders*. Las Vegas, NV: International Imports, 1985.

———. *The Modern Spellbook: The Magical Uses of Herbs*. Las Vegas, NV: International Imports, 1974.

Scheub, Harold. *A Dictionary of African Mythology: The Mythmaker as Storyteller*. Oxford: Oxford University Press, 2000.

Snow, Loudell F. *Walkin' Over Medicine*. Boulder, San Francisco, Oxford: Westview Press, 1993.

Some, Malidoma Patrice. *The Healing Wisdom of Africa: Finding Life Purpose Through Nature, Ritual and Community*. New York: Jeremy P. Tarcher/Putnam, 1999.

Thompson, Robert Farris. *Flash of the Spirit: African and Afro-American Art and Philosophy*. New York: Vintage Books, 1983.

Umeh, J.A. *After God is Dibla: Igbo Cosmology, Divination & Sacred Science in Nigeria, Volume Two*. London: Karnak House, 1999.

United Plant Savers. "UpS 'At-Risk' & 'To Watch' Lists." *Planting the Future. http://united-plantsavers.org*

US Department of Homeland Security, FEMA. "Residential Smoking Fires and Casualties." *Topical Fire Research* Series 5, issue 5 (June 2005). *http://www.usfa.fema.gov/*

Van Wyk, Ben-Erik and Nigel Gericke. *People's Plants—A Guide to Useful Plants of Southern Africa*. Pretoria, South Africa: Briza Publications, 2000.

Voeks, Robert A. *Sacred Leaves of Candomble: African Magic, Medicine, and Religion in Brazil*. Austin, TX: University of Texas Press, 1997.

Walker, Barbara. *The Woman's Encyclopedia of Myths and Secrets*. Edison, NJ: Castle Books, 1991.

Weil, Andrew. *Spontaneous Healing: How to Discover and Enhance Your Body's Natural Ability to Maintain and Heal Itself*. New York: Ballantine Books and Fawcett Columbine, 1995.

Westmacott, Richard. *African-American Gardens and Yards in the Rural South*. Knoxville, TN: University of Tennessee Press, 1992.

Worwood, Valerie Ann. *The Complete Book of Essential Oils and Aromatherapy*. Novato, CA: New World Library, 1991.

Zak, Victoria. *20,000 Uses of Tea*. New York: Dell Publishing, A Division of Random House, 1999.

Index

About the Author

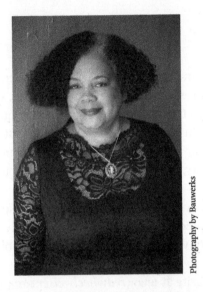

Stephanie Rose Bird is a painter and the author of several bestselling books on earth spirituality, Hoodoo, and anthropology, including *Sticks, Stones, Roots, and Bones, 365 Days of Hoodoo, Light, Bright, and Damned Near White,* and *African American Magick.* Bird, who holds a BFA cum laude and an MFA, is a devotee of the Divinely Feminine. She is an Elder, Priestess, magick-maker and keeper of the spiritual wisdom of her indigenous African ancestors. Her work centers around the nexus of earth wisdom and the legacy of Black cultural heritage. Find her at *www.stephanierosebird.com* and follow her on Instagram @s.r.bird

To Our Readers